THE HOSPITAL
REVOLUTION

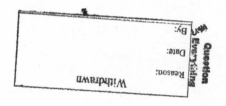

Withdrawn

Reason:

Date:

By:

Everykiding

Question

D1421674

THE HOSPITAL REVOLUTION

DOCTORS REVEAL THE CRISIS ENGULFING BRITAIN'S HEALTH SERVICE

JOHN RIDDINGTON YOUNG et al

Aided and Abetted by PETER TOMLIN

metro

Published by Metro, an imprint of John Blake Publishing Ltd,
3 Bramber Court, 2 Bramber Road,
London W14 9PB, England

www.blake.co.uk

First published in paperback in 2008

ISBN 978 1 84454 595 7

British Library Cataloguing-in-Publication Data:

A catalogue record for this book is available from the British Library.

Design by www.envydesign.co.uk

Printed in the UK by CPI William Clowes Beccles NR34 7TL

1 3 5 7 9 10 8 6 4 2

Papers used by John Blake Publishing are natural, recyclable products made from
wood grown in sustainable forests. The manufacturing processes conform to the
environmental regulations of the country of origin.

Every attempt has been made to contact the relevant copyright-holders, but some were
unobtainable. We would be grateful if the appropriate people could contact us.

To all those who *work* in our NHS Hospitals
We emphasise the word *work*

John Riddington Young

JRY is the Senior Consultant Surgeon at the North Devon District Hospital, where he has worked (when not suspended) since 1981. His particular sub-speciality interest in E.N.T. is the sexual aspects of the nose (a field in which he says there is little competition)! He obtained a Master of Philosophy degree from the Open University (Department of the History of Science and Technology) and graduated in Brussels in 2000 for a research thesis entitled *Medical Ideas in English Poetry to the End of the Seventeenth Century.*

He has published other books on historical research, the first being a study of the *Inns and Taverns of Old Norwich* when he was a houseman (1972). More recently he co-authored a book on the history of otolaryngology, *Offbeat Otolaryngology*. Other obscure books written by him include an illustrated book on Devon Church History and a short book on (Devon) Military History.

He has always had military connections and was the Commanding Officer of 211 (Wessex) Field Hospital based in Plymouth. He is still on the Army List and holds an active rank of substantive Colonel. Since being a junior doctor, he has continuously been a staunch supporter of the St. John Ambulance Brigade and is an Officer in the Most Venerable Order of the Hospital of Saint John of Jerusalem.

Over the past few years, he has raised over £13,000 for local charities by undertaking sponsored long distance walks. Just before the first (legitimate) Gulf War in 2002, he also raised over £1600 for the Army Benevolent Fund by having his moustache shaved off! He lists his hobbies as long distance walking, fishing, shooting, making stained-glass windows, cabinet-making, woodcarving, Punch and Judy, growing prize-winning Sweet Peas, British Bulldogs and Arabic calligraphy.

The Second Author

The second author is also a Consultant Surgeon working in an NHS hospital, but unlike JRY has not yet been suspended and would therefore like to keep his name undisclosed, since he realises what a traumatic process this can be. To shroud his identity, too many details of his curriculum vitae cannot be revealed, but he is willing to divulge certain facts: he is a former junior mixed infant and grammar school scholarship boy; his hero is Dreyfus and his hobbies include playing the grand piano, ballroom dancing and correcting misuse of the apostrophe.

Peter Tomlin

Dr Tomlin has no such qualms as the aforesaid co-author about possible suspension because he undoubtedly knows more about the suspension of doctors in the NHS than anyone else in the world and anyway, he is now retired. He was on the Parliamentary Working Party on the Suspension of Doctors with Baroness Young. He now currently spends most of his busy retirement fighting the corner of his suspended colleagues since he is the Secretary of the Study Group of Suspended Doctors. He was formerly a Consultant Anaesthetist in the Midlands.

PREFACE

The authors, who are all hospital consultants, feel that the layman has no awareness of the intense internecine power struggle that is going on in hospitals between the medical staff and the administrators. The public are amazed to learn that in most hospitals, these administrators are paid higher salaries than the most senior and experienced doctors. Very few lay people are aware of the minimal academic qualifications and lack of any proper Civil Service training of these so-called managers and are incredulous of the excessive power that they wield. The book is designed principally to inform the public of the bizarre situation in which poorly trained non-qualified staff, who are despised by many doctors and respected by none, run our hospitals. Many true anecdotes are told of their unbelievable incompetence. The premise is made that the NHS would improve if all these managers were removed, because not only do they do no good, but also they exert a definite negative influence, particularly on the morale of the people who actually work in hospitals, which never before has been so incredibly low.

Although the book is aimed at the layman who is interested in healthcare and politics, doctors too will be delighted to read this work. They are tired of being the whipping boy for the nation's health shortcomings. Their mistakes are widely publicised – their hard work is inevitably neglected. This book restores the balance and is the required 'tonic' for any doctor who is beginning to feel that the job may not be worth the candle. From the profession's ancient origins to possible future developments, relations with other professions and workers and much more, all are analysed with incisive wit and aplomb.

The authors would like to acknowledge all the help they received from PJT without whose help it would have been quite impossible to write the last chapter.

CONTENTS

In which the authors examine the evolution of the NHS, paying particular attention to the complex ethical concepts which drove it for many years, but which now sadly have been forcibly changed. They describe a 'Revolution' in which the benign self-regulation, which had slowly evolved since the time of Hippocrates, has been substituted in recent years for commercial and political ideologies by successive Governments of both political parties.

CHAPTER 2: MORALE

In which the authors examine the importance and origin of morale and goodwill, which always were the major currency of the overburdened, underpaid health service workers. Attention is drawn to the reasons how and why morale is now at such an all-time nadir that doctors are leaving the NHS in droves.

CHAPTER 3: LIONS DRIVEN BY DONKEYS

In which the administrators are shown in a number of true anecdotes to be inept and incompetent buffoons. The authors outline the political changes since 1985 that have given rise to an explosion in the numbers of these people. The absolute absence of any proper training or management structure is described, and the complete lack of any leadership skills that has caused the low morale in hospitals is presented.

CHAPTER 4: DUTY, PRIVILEGE AND RESPONSIBILITY   87

In which the ethical concepts introduced in the first chapter are expanded. Professionalism and the personal nature of the doctor-patient relationship that existed in the early days of the NHS are contrasted with impersonal managerialism and the market-place mentality forced on doctors in the 1980s. Inside stories of incredible recent managerial gaffes in Luton, Plymouth and South Molton.

CHAPTER 5: FEES AND REMUNERATION   111

After a brief historical resumé including how doctors were paid in medieval times, the bizarre story is revealed of how Corkscrew Charlie and Aneurin Bevan decided how much they were worth at the inception of the NHS. Few laymen realise that the non-qualified hospital executives get substantially bigger salaries than doctors. The Quisling doctors who, driven by financial incentives and their own avarice for lucre vile, have turned their backs on their professional colleagues and have joined the ranks of the administrators are also presented.

CHAPTER 6: PEOPLE ARE MORE IMPORTANT THAN PLACES   133

In which more almost unbelievable anecdotes of mismanagement and incompetent bungling illustrate eloquently how morale has been destroyed and all the working hospital staff from porters to consultants have been made to feel utterly unvalued.

CHAPTER 7: THE NEW LANGUAGE   155

In which 'Political Correctness' is defined as the incorrect use of English and also in which the authors explore how hospital managers try to alter the meaning of words such as 'colleague' and 'trust' for their own political expediency.

CHAPTER 8: DISCIPLINING HOSPITAL DOCTORS IN THE NATIONAL HEALTH SERVICE

In which Dr Peter Tomlin shows how the NHS managers put themselves beyond the law. Incredible revelations are disclosed about the unlawful measures hospital managers have used to humiliate hospital doctors who would not toe the line. The anecdotes in this chapter are frightening and unbelievable.

CONCLUSION

In which some clear, controversial and positive suggestions are made to stem the incoming tide of despair. The administrators are likened to a cancer which is slowly killing the Service and the only treatment is to remove it. The hundreds of untrained and incompetent bureaucrats should be replaced by a few retired senior consultants, who have experience of the hospital and a primary humanitarian ethic and the respect of the work force. With the expulsion of the Executives and their replacement by someone whom they could respect, all hospital workers (even the few administrators in the new proposed system!) would once again feel valued. With that leadership, morale, which has been missing for so long, would return to our hospitals and the massive exodus of highly qualified professionals would cease. Some might even come back! The unbelievable cruelty of the present suspension system must be exposed to the public as an example of the waste (and the contumely) of the managers. It must then be removed forever and replaced by a fair and just system.

PROLEGOMENON

What is wrong with our National Health Service? What has happened to it? Why is it in such a plight? It once used to be the envy of less happier lands but now most of the people who work in it will tell you it is in a sorry and dejected state.

The NHS itself is clearly very sick.

But why is the morale of its doctors and nurses at such an all time low? Why are these professionals taking early retirement in such hitherto unprecedented numbers?

Recently, surgeons received a circular from the President of the Royal College of Surgeons of England in which he said that the morale of colleagues throughout the country is the lowest that it has been during most of their lives and that 'frustration and despondency is at an alarming all time high'.

Hospitals were once, despite their burden of human suffering, happy places to work. Why have they now become depressing and doleful places in which to spend one's working week? Why can't doctors (and nurses) wait to retire?

The reason is that in the past they felt *valued.* Now they certainly do not! Their salaries in fact used to be lower, but they felt that a very great part of their job satisfaction was from the *esprit de corps* of their fellow hospital workers and they had a true sense that society in general actually appreciated the work they did. It is not only the medical and nursing professionals, but others who actually follow some useful occupations in hospitals – lab technicians, pharmacists, radiologists, hospital porters, telephonists, kitchen staff and ward cleaners; they will all tell you that over the last dozen or so years things have drastically changed for the worse in our once wonderful National Health Service and not one of them now feels that their essential contributions are valued by their employers.

There has been a very definite revolution.

But who has caused that revolution? It has certainly not been the medics themselves: they have been too busy working!

That revolution is solely and exclusively due to the arrival of hordes of totally unqualified administrators into the hospitals. This was a politically motivated idea dreamed up by Government.

When your authors started to work for the NHS, the old hospital phone books showed four administrators (on the back page); now (on the front page) there starts a list of over one hundred phone numbers marked 'Management'. (They might have changed their name but they certainly want you to realize they have arrived.) For an easy comparison over the same period, the number of consultants has only just about doubled!

In the past there used to be the Matron (for Nursing and Ward Matters) and a harassed looking chap in a shabby suit called the Hospital Secretary. There was also a Treasurer and the Lady Almoner (currently called the Social Worker). Now there are scores of them. The stereotypes now are women in badly fitting tight suits (often carrying millboards or stacks of paper to give the impression that they are busy) and a quite a few more harassed looking men running after them. This is probably because these fellows are now bossed about by the women, who are in the definite majority. They don't even like to call themselves 'administrators' nowadays; they prefer the term 'managers'. Doctors still insist on calling them by their old title however, which implies that they only exist to administrate the requirements of the medical consultants who have a clear and imperative supremacy in the hospital hierarchy.

Where did these myriads of middle management, often with no previous experience of the NHS, come from? During the eighties, most private industry was getting rid of large numbers of middle-tier managers for sound economic reasons. One supposes that all these redundant second-raters had to go somewhere. At a time when there were many failed managers who had been kicked out by industry and were looking for jobs, the NHS (which by definition had always been a charity) took on hundreds of administrators, some of whom had previously worked for chain stores or bus companies. But doctors, nurses (and most other hospital *workers*) aren't quite the same as shop-assistants and bus conductors; for one thing doctors don't do things such as going on strike (like car-workers and dockers): if we did, our patients would suffer. Unlike hospital administrators, doctors actually do put patients first. Most physicians try to form relationships with their patients and genuinely care about them; their wellbeing is paramount. This is clearly not the perception of the managers who are accountants and it seems try to run their trusts like chain stores.

The influx of these civil servants into the hospital scene by Government was almost certainly financially motivated, but it does not even seem to have made any impression on the finances. Before they came, when hospitals were happy places, everyone always used to grumble about under-funding but got the job done, and at the end of the day there was a financial deficit. Now the main difference seems to be that nothing gets done, morale has been devastated and at the end of the day the hospital is in an even greater debt! The grumbling of course still goes on.

They have also made monumental mistakes in their utter incompetence with respect to their attempts at the regulation and control of Doctors. This had hitherto always been a self-governing process which had evolved over many years and was mainly administered by other doctors in the same hospital or the General Medical Council (GMC). It had absolutely nothing at all to do with financial considerations but was based on old fashioned Hippocratic principles and wholly concerned with patient care. This self regulation has now been completely replaced by these power-mad bureaucrats, whose main drive in life seems to be fuelled not even by monetary considerations but almost unbelievably appears to be a spiteful jealousy that they are not themselves medically qualified – so they try to humiliate those who are. This has led to a complete lack of trust and confidence in administrative support staff ('managers') and a feeling (as a senior surgeon put it to one of the authors very recently) that you always have to 'watch your back.'

Thomas Jefferson said that, 'When the People fear the Government, that is Tyranny; When the Government fears the People, that is Democracy.' The NHS administrators are certainly tyrannical. Big Brother (in the Orwellian rather than the Channel 4 sense) is always watching you and eager to find fault and throw you out of the place! What a terrible environment in which to work!

Small wonder that doctors want to take ever earlier retirement. They no longer feel valued and cannot trust their employers.

A surgeon who had been suspended and sent home from work in 2006 for something the television news described at the time as 'insignificant', met one of his old patients in the foyer as he was being escorted to the main door of the hospital by the policeman. Understandably, he told the old man that he never intended coming back to work in a place which held his services in such low esteem. 'Don't give in!' said the old fellow to the surgeon, 'You saved my life! Your patients appreciate you! You work for us, you don't work for them!'

The old man had hit the nail on the head. Physicians and surgeons never for one minute think that they work for anyone but their patients. They would retire even earlier if they actually thought that they worked for their incompetent administrators. When discussing this perceived lack of worth by our employers, a consultant orthopaedic surgeon suggested that perhaps it is because they realise that they themselves are so utterly useless that the administrators do not value anyone else in the hospital.

One amazing fact is that the administrators honestly believe themselves to have the authority to be the *Leaders* of the hospital and yet they have no powers of leadership whatsoever and command no respect amongst the doctors (quite the reverse). They receive extremely high salaries *often substantially higher than the surgeons who work throughout the night in the operating theatres.*

The internecine hatred, which exists between the administrators and medically qualified staff is not generally realized by the public who still cling to the old assumption that doctors are still in charge of the important decisions made in the running of our hospitals.

It is the firm belief of the authors that all the problems that presently exist within a once excellent service can be blamed fairly and squarely on these officious officials, who of course, have absolutely no medical qualifications whatsoever. We would go further and suggest that were they *all* removed (yes, every last one!), the overall result would be an improvement. Morale would rocket to unprecedented levels, hospitals would become happy places to work again and billions of pounds would become available to be put to much better use: for example, the actual clinical care of patients, rather than the salaries of thousands of unnecessary managers. We would hasten to point out that we are not actually suggesting that every last one should get the sack (however wonderful a picture this presents to the doctors of Britain) but we use this beautiful hypothetical scenario to emphasise just how expensive and pernicious they have become to our healthcare service. Perhaps one or two could be retained at each larger hospital under the supervision of a Medical Superintendent.

The sad truth of the matter however is that even a small reduction in their numbers is never likely to take place. The people in charge of hiring and firing employees in the NHS are the administrators themselves and they are hardly likely to sack each other.

They certainly do not like to be reminded of Dr Albert Schweitzer, the famous African missionary physician and Nobel Peace Prize winner. He was a brilliant theologian, gifted musician and dedicated doctor and should be a shining example to us all. This great genius wrote many scholarly tracts and set up hospitals and leper colonies in Equatorial Africa. He once said that:

You can easily run hospitals without administrators; it is easy and I have done it many times. You can also run hospitals without laboratories and X-rays; it is not so easy, but I have done it occasionally. You can even run hospitals without qualified nurses; it is extremely difficult, but I have done it on a few occasions. But you cannot run hospitals without doctors!

There again, Albert Schweitzer was a doctor.

CHAPTER 1

THE PROFESSION OF MEDICINE

Limited Resources, Unlimited Demands

A doctor's work (according to Rudyard Kipling):

> The world has long ago decided that you have no working hours that anybody is bound to respect; that nothing but extreme bodily illness will excuse you in its eyes from refusing to help a man who thinks he may need your help at any hour of the day or night. That in all times of flood, fire, famine, plague, pestilence, battle, murder or sudden death, it will be required of you that you report for duty, go on duty at once, and remain on duty, until your strength fails you or your conscience relieves you, whichever may be the longer period.

Mind you, Rudyard Kipling had some very strange notions about medicine. On 15 December 1928, in his 64th year, he addressed the Royal Society of Medicine in London on the subject of: 'Healing by the Stars – a Plea for a Return to Astrology'.

The public's attitude to medicine and healthcare has become very demanding – in some cases unrealistically so. It has got to the stage where many medical people feel the force of Kipling's words, in a context that the poet did not envisage. They feel themselves on a moving treadmill, which they cannot get off and which is getting out of control. Yet, despite ever more effort, the public's demands remain unsatisfied. Is this the fault, or responsibility, of the profession? When the NHS was formed in 1948 there was some naive political optimism that unrestricted free medical attention would become a self-limiting expense. However, the founder of the Service, Aneurin Bevan himself, did foresee the inevitability of unsatisfied demands on his new service. He said: 'We will never have all we need; this service must always be growing, changing and improving; it must always appear to be inadequate.'

One of his successors was the great intellect, scholar, and fearless speaker of the truth, Enoch Powell (Tory) Minister of Health from 1960 to 1963 (and in the opinion of quite a few of his generation of consultants and GPs, the best one we have ever had)[1]. His erudite rhetoric and convincing eloquence were legendary, and it was he who coined the phrase 'Limited Resources but unlimited Demands' for the exigencies of the NHS. In his book *Medicine and Politics* he wrote:

> Every advance in medical science creates new needs that did not exist until the means of meeting them came into existence ... there is virtually no limit to the amount of medical care an individual is capable of absorbing ...

[1] John Enoch Powell MA (Cantab) MBE PC (1912–1988) Professor of Greek at the University of Sydney 1937 joined the Royal Warwickshire Regiment as a private soldier in 1939 and was commissioned in 1940, becoming a Brigadier-General by 1944. Member of Parliament 1950–1987.

improvement in expectation of survival results in lives that demand further medical care.

A Dinner of Herbs, Where Love Is[2]

The authors have a friend whose wife broke her leg whilst on holiday in Italy and was admitted to a tiny convent hospital there, which was run by nuns. She paints a picture straight out of *Heidi* of a small ward with its whitewashed walls and scrubbed pine floorboards. There was a bowl of fresh alpine flowers on the table and a flaking painted crucifix on the wall – and four spartan beds. The place was run by a handful of nuns – only one of whom could speak English. She was not sure how many of them had nursing qualifications, but there were lots of helpers from the village who acted as nursing auxiliaries. There were no curtains. The beds were hard, the mattresses thin and the pillows lumpy. The relatives of the other three patients, who also brought in fresh bed linen for her, often made the beds. Everybody was terribly kind and fussed over her. They brought in food for her and little presents, but they couldn't understand her, nor she them, and they got terribly worried when they thought she wanted anything[3].

After a few days, the insurance company sorted out the air ambulance, and the bed-ridden patient was given an impromptu leaving party before being repatriated back home. She was sorry, in a way, to leave them because they had been so kind to her, but she was looking forward to getting back to a 'proper hospital'. She was terribly reassured when she was wheeled into the

---

[2] 'Better a dinner of herbs where love is than a stalled ox and hatred therewith,' Proverbs 15.17. This is from the authorised version. Matthew's Bible (1535) states: 'Better a mess of potage with love than a fat ox with evil will.'

[3] One of the few words they did (luckily) understand was 'pee-pee'.

District General Hospital and saw the comfortable looking beds with curtains round them. 'Luxury' she thought, at last she'd be able to have a *pee-pee* in private! At last she had *arrived* and could now receive first class nursing care for her full recovery.

So much for her expectations.

When the moment came, and she used the state of the art electric push-button, flash-a-light gadget on her bedside console – no one came. Three nurses were looking after the thirty patients on the ward. She couldn't even attract an auxiliary. At least in the convent she could always find a willing helper, even if it was one who could speak no English. They had been sympathetic and helpful and somehow she had felt safe in the little ward high up in the Italian mountains. She had known she was in kind loving hands. Now in the UK, in our wonderful National Health Service, she felt alone and vulnerable[4].

A leading article in the *Lancet* once summed it up well: 'Of the many ways of judging a medical service, none perhaps is more valid than to measure it by the trust it inspires in those whom it serves.' However, that was written in 1958. In those days things were very different. But a Revolution was about to take place.

A dear friend, a retired Consultant venereologist from Sheffield, and a Glaswegian, told us when we announced our intention of writing this book that its pages would be stained by the tears of his generation of doctors, now retired, who came out of the Army in 1946, and were not particularly optimistic about the new NHS. When it arrived, they felt that their wartime Service

---

[4]Some nurses can be too helpful. A colleague was summoned to a ward at night by a distraught student nurse. A patient was in 'status epilepticus' (permanent epileptic fitting). After dragging himself out of bed he reached the ward and found the cubicle; luckily he was able to reassure the young Nightingale that the patient was simply masturbating.

had been a sort of rehearsal for the new State medical system, and he said that, it worked so 'beautifully' at first, and continued to work very well for many years ... until 'managers' came along, that's when he personally reckoned the rot set in, and the Revolution began. Let us explain.

The Revolution

Edmund Burke, the politician who condemned the French Jacobins and wrote *Reflections on the Revolution in France* in 1790 suggested in a letter to their National Assembly: 'Make the Revolution a parent of settlement, and not the nursery of future revolutions.' The actual date of the Hospital Revolution is open to debate: it certainly did not come overnight: it crept up on us like an insidious cancer, but we are all very sure that it has taken place! It is an interesting exercise to ask one's colleagues when they consider the rot first set into the hospitals. Those to the right of centre blame Harold Wilson's Minister of Health, Mrs Barbara Castle[5] (1974–76) and her attempts to remove the élitist status of doctors (and more especially nurses). Quite a few say it was with Mrs Thatcher's 'internal market' reforms of April Fool's Day 1991; some go back to the demise of the Hospital Secretary and his replacement with administrators, who rapidly set about demonstrating

[5]Although she did *act* as Minister of Health, her Labour predecessor Crossman (who took over the post after the Labour general election victory of 1968) had for some reason changed the title to 'Secretary of State for Social Services'. One of your authors, who is from Sheffield, remembers a tale about this Lancastrian redhead. A new pub had been built in Sheffield on the site of an older one called 'The Castle'. Because of Sheffield's long association with the Labour Party (hence its nickname 'The People's Republic of South Yorkshire') it was thought that it would be a nice gesture to ask the titian-haired Minister to open it. The story that went around at the time was that, when invited to perform the opening ceremony she asked for a fee, and, as a result, the idea was abandoned. Whatever the facts, the pub was not renamed 'The Castle', but 'The Red Cow'. They have a sharp sense of humour in Sheffield!

Parkinson's Fourth Law[6]; others believe it was when the administrators shed that description (a senior colleague with a feeling for language, who has since joined the majority, was wont to remind them that that word meant to minister unto) and became managers[7]. There are all sorts of suggestions, but no one, not even the most traitorous, back-stabbing, 'Doctor Turncoat' (Medical Director) answers the question by saying: 'What do you mean? There is no problem!'

Some colleagues old enough to remember it, reckon that the Revolution started some twenty-five years before Maggie Thatcher's attempts to bring the market place into the hospitals (shedding the political embarrassment of government responsibility) with the inception of budget-holding Trusts and fund-holders in 1990. They blame the Salmon Report of 1966.

One of the authors of this book well remembers Hospital Matrons and he has no doubt at all that they were the *one* key figure in the hospitals, before the Revolution. They ate hospital administrators for breakfast (and quite often junior consultants for lunch!). In order to destabilize the hospital hierarchy, it would be necessary to 'take out' Matron first. That was the Labour Party's strategy: destroy the nurses first and then take on the doctors in a second offensive. The elimination of Matron as the key-figure was the first move and this was brought about by

---

[6]The number of people in any working group tends to increase regardless of the amount of work to be done.

[7]Of course, only obsequious toadies ever call them managers; most doctors don't even realise they no longer like being called administrators anyway. An added little advantage of using the former term is that the correct female form is *administratrix* (see *Fowler: Modern English Usage* for a full description of whether or not to use the plural *administratrixes* or *administratrices*; no collective noun is given – your authors suggest coven.)

Brian Salmon, director of the caterers J. Lyons (and nephew of Sir Keith Joseph, then Minister of Health). He made an excellent job of destroying the structure of the nursing hierarchy. In 1966 the Salmon Report kicked out the Matrons, demoralised the Ward Sisters, and forced the nurses into the arms of the Trade Unions; this was seen by many doctors (and nurses) as the first nail in the coffin of professionalism for the nurse.

Prior to the establishment of the NHS, the British Hospital System was a traditional charitable institution built up over many decades to produce something that might have been born of the old-fashioned Victorian values of the 1832 Poor Law Act. Perhaps because of, rather than in spite of, that sense of dedication of its staff, it had the certain, firm and undoubted respect, and therefore support, of the public it served. It had absorbed, in the idiosyncratic British way, Aneurin Bevan's change in its funding (and in its 'ownership') into its Christian ethos, to become the envy of the First World.

The poor nurses then, were the first casualties. They were a soft target. Their *esprit de corps* was crushed. Their attractive uniforms were condemned as élitist and substituted by overalls, to which they could attach a name badge rather like at supermarkets with just their first name on, rather than Staff Nurse Smith or the like[8]. The usual (still quoted) platitudes about 'bringing in changes to keep up with the technological progress

---

[8]It is interesting to note that at least one consultant surgeon – who used to write to one of the plain-clothes harridans in charge of the nurses at his hospital complaining that nurses, now depleted of their aprons, cuffs and caps (he didn't even mention the black *seamed* stockings!) had begun to look like dinner ladies in their Jaycloth overalls – now tells us that he has had to revise his criticism: the dinner ladies at his hospital have been 'privatised' and started to wear nice frilly white aprons, white cuffs and smart little caps … he adds sadly that they don't wear the stockings yet!

in medicine' were quoted for this[9]. They were the first to be pushed into seeking more money and shorter working hours in lieu of recognition, support and respect, which explains the escalating cost of the Service.

The hospitals did in fact have administrators, or at least *an* Administrator. He was called the Hospital Secretary, because he was responsible for the secretariat: he was usually an amiable cove in a crumpled suit who did his utmost to help the doctors and nurses make the best use of their finite resources, and often left the door of his office open to show his availability to staff to come to him with their problems. The ones which the authors remember all smoked heavily, but were courteous and respectful. They did not suffer from delusions of grandeur. They knew their place in the order of things and were happy with it. They knew they could never even start to do the doctors' work (let alone the nurses') and did not have a chip on their shoulder about their obvious subordinate status.

Hospitals were, for all their burden of human misery, satisfying places to work in, and in those days the Hospital Secretary would even be welcomed as part of the hospital cricket team. Everybody would pull together for the good of the patients. What on earth has happened to produce the embittered internecine divisions that now crush morale, accelerate compassion fatigue, and lead physically healthy but bitterly disillusioned colleagues to take early retirement in unprecedented numbers? What caused the amiable chap in the

---

[9]Repeating a lie often enough usually causes it to be accepted as a truth. Many people (including some doctors) believe that a swan is strong enough to break a man's leg with a blow from its wing. Others are still convinced that the only animal that cannot swim is the pig – because it cuts its own throat with its sharp little trotters! The authors refute both these oft-repeated myths as well.

unpressed suit to metamorphose into dozens of top-salaried vicious ex-accountants, ex-businessmen and ex-nurses seemingly hell-bent on self-aggrandizement at the cost of our once wonderful Hospital Service?[10] The Victorians had a great awareness of precedence; and referred to upstarts as *parvenus*[11].

At Last, an 84-Hour Week

One of your authors, dear reader, was working as a house-surgeon in Doncaster at the time when Mrs Barbara Castle took up the cause of some of the more vociferous overworked underpaid hospital doctors in training, who, for a year or two, spent many hours in the hospital wards and nearly as many sleeping in the hospital in order to be available to patients, with very little time off[12]. Mrs. Castle instituted the revolutionary new eighty-four hour availability week, with alternate nights off, for these highly qualified apprentices in their twenties (doubling the numbers needed). Of course, not all our chiefs were in favour of these 'namby-pamby milk-sop reforms': they had worked hard to

---

[10]History is not without parallels: 'The artisans' objection to the capitalism which, in the early nineteenth century, increasingly denied the moral economy which gave the trades their modest but respected place, was not so much to working masters, whom they had long known, or to machinery as such, which could be seen as an extension of hand tools, but to the capitalist seen as an unproductive and parasitic middleman.' Hobsbawm 1983.

[11]From the past participle of the intransitive French verb *parvenir* – to arrive. Doctors trace their professional origins back to Hippocrates on the island of Kos in 460BC. Secular nurses' origins, beyond the arrival on the scene of Miss Nightingale over 100 years ago, may best have a discreet veil drawn over them, suffice to say that they were certainly members of a very ancient (perhaps even the oldest) profession.

[12]In earlier times they used to send little children down coalmines: in the opinion of the other author, this would have been preferable to working as a house surgeon at the Doncaster Royal Infirmary.

gain their experience and they didn't see how anybody could learn their trade unless they saw enough cases, nor, perhaps more importantly, how youngsters who had prolonged their self-centred adolescence through five or six years in medical school, could learn to subordinate their interests to those of their patients without a baptism of fire (and there was certainly a degree of truth in their views – anachronistic as they may seem in today's society). Mrs Castle compromised by allowing anyone who spent more than the new eighty-four hour week on duty to get a form signed by their consultant, and they would be paid extra for the hours that they had put in.

One of your authors can quite clearly remember a Sir Lancelot Spratt type gathering everybody together and saying very definitely that nobody need bother filling in these forms, because they would *certainly* not be signed! Your author hastens to add that this surgeon was a caring, dedicated man who was himself willing to work every hour that God sent, and didn't see why fellow professionals should start to fill in overtime slips (like a factory worker) for learning to practise a vocation which should be considered a privilege in itself. Many of his colleagues (who some thought to be more enlightened) signed the controversial slips, and it became commonplace, and for far less than eighty-four hours a week. Many colleagues saw this as the thin end of a wedge driven between 'masters' and 'employers'.

It was the start of the slippery slope away from professionalism. We were no longer high-minded members of a noble profession with philanthropic Hippocratic ideals, dedicated to the patient whose needs were paramount, with pay of secondary importance (in some hospitals it was called a 'stipend' – the salary paid to a clergyman). Our rot had started, and we had begun lowering our standards and our commitment to those of a garage mechanic[13]. It could justifiably be argued that we had started to prostitute ourselves[14].

The authors do not believe this to have been the start of the Revolution, but view it as an important incident undermining the ethics of doctors, and a factor in setting the scene for further changes. A few years later some of the junior doctors showed the country that they had prostituted themselves utterly when they abandoned their patients altogether and went on strike for more pay. Left wing cynics said that Mrs Castle and her cronies had succeeded in discrediting the middle-class doctors, and shown them in their true colours as money-grabbing capitalists who put their purse before their patients (and the authors must sadly admit that there *have* always been *some* – like lecherous clergy or crooked politicians) but it may be truer to say that she had kick-started the degradation of a conscientious and self-regulating artisan class, with a formal apprenticeship system, and craft rules of dedication to the service of the sick, into a unionised skilled labour force in perpetual conflict with their capitalist, and would-be monopolist 'employer'.

Doctors in General Practice in 1948 wisely, or luckily, managed to avoid becoming 'employees'. They rightly insisted that they worked for their patients, no matter who footed the bill, and remained (for the most part) dedicated, hard working, modestly rewarded, and respected members of their communities. They were, however, unable to avoid the increasing trivialisation of their workload, as their surgeries became filled with the submerged

---

[13]We do not, of course, include our own mechanics in this! We have the utmost respect for their competence and professional manner.

[14]The word 'prostitute' is derived from the Latin words *pro* and *statuo* meaning 'to place before' – one's profit before one's principles.

tenth of the population who learned that doctors were the helpless gateway to freeloading on the new welfare state, and subsequent to this, the doctor's job satisfaction plummeted[15].

Cogwheel and the Stasi

'Cogwheel' was a buzzword invented by the administrators in 1967[16]. It was an attempt to upgrade the minimal contribution of the Drain Sniffers, which is the derisive term used by those doctors who practise medicine for those who administrate; (the term takes its origin from the time when the old Medical Officers of Health appeared to concern themselves mainly with dirt, sanitation and the lavatory). Those older readers who nostalgically can remember black and white television episodes of *Dr Finlay's Casebook* might well recall with affection Dr Snoddy, the MOH for Tannoch Brae, and his little glass phials containing specimens of faeces and sputum. In fact, Dr Snoddy and the appointment of MOH were relics of Sir Edwin Chadwick's Public Health Act of 1848.

Chadwick was a barrister and believed (quite rightly) that effective sanitation, improved drainage and water closets for all, would radically improve the health of the nation. His report[i] was mainly concerned with sanitary reforms, but also separated public health doctors (the drain sniffers) from the rest of clinical[17] medicine (a schism which still persists).

In the pre-NHS days, the non-teaching hospitals had a Medical

---

[15]See *Honour a Physician* by Richard Asher.

[16]In 1966, Sir George Godber, a Chief Medical Officer, established a working party of the MoH and the Joint Consultants Committee of the BMA to try to involve doctors in administration. The first report in 1967 was immediately called *Cogwheel* because of the motif on the cover.

[17]From *clinos* Greek: bed.

Superintendent, who was medically qualified and did a part-time consultant job in the hospital, but also attended to administrative matters such as disciplinary matters of junior colleagues, the health problems of hospital staff and liaison with the Board. It was generally reckoned by our older colleagues that it was a useful and well-respected job, and if 'a prestigious consultant with knowledge and instincts for management'[18] held the post, the hospital would be well run. The reader might reflect that in the United States of America, a country no stranger to efficiency and market economics, this is the pattern often still found[19]. In fact the US Health system is generally held to be the worst in the First World.

The most odious part of the Cogwheel document is to be found in paragraph 33; it is the conclusion that: 'In the face of the need for collective thinking, there is nothing to be gained by the re-establishment of the old-style full time medical superintendent.'

Happily, the thinly disguised philosophy of Cogwheel (which was written by a drain sniffer, Sir George Godber, with drain sniffers in mind) never fooled anyone and so never took off. Perhaps another reason was because of the symbol, which was used to promote it. It was a bit like a Hindu mandala, although a lot of the older doctors, who were around at the time say that they were like three swastikas, but perhaps this is because they associate it with an administration that seemed to be getting more and more like the Gestapo[20]. It might have even been around this time that some disaffected doctors adopted the title 'Stasi' for the administrators. This was the common

---

[18]We borrow this phrase from the Enthoven Report 1985 (vi).

[19]The authors caution the reader not to make *too* much of this – in that country McDonalds is after all considered to be a restaurant.

[20]Contraction of *Geheime Staatspolizei* ('secret state police'), the official secret police of Nazi Germany.

term (rather like Nazi) for the German *Staatssicherheitsdienst* and fitted in well as a descriptive term for the Administration. Like many police states, East Germany (Deutsche Demokratische Republik or DDR) was full of euphemisms, double-speak and downright lies. Its actual name of 'democratic' is an example, and is not unlike the NHS use of the word 'Trust'. Anyway, the Stasi were the Security Police and if any reader wants to know how life was between the construction of the Berlin Wall (1961) and its fall (1989), then the authors recommend the excellent award-winning film 'The Lives of Others' (*Das Leben der Anderen*)[21].

The Stasi was not in itself large in terms of numbers, but was very well equipped. Its strength lay not only in its ability to fulfil its aim 'to know everything' but also to intimidate the population and recruit those who, for the promise of future preferment, would inform on others. Is something beginning to sound familiar? Usually they had no difficulty in recruitment – people with a grudge would approach the authorities with information which they felt they 'had to bring to someone's attention'. Often the victim would have no idea what he had been accused of, or even that an accusation had taken place – life would slowly get more difficult for him, and, not surprisingly, sometimes better for the Stasi's 'helper'. The reader will no doubt notice hereinafter that this pet-name (Stasi) will be adopted from time to time for administrators.

---

[21]This film was released by Sony in the UK in April 2007 with English subtitles. Since some of our American friends are unaccustomed to subtitles and do not seem to be able to watch a film and read at the same time (a recent US President was reported to be unable to chew gum and fart simultaneously) there are evidently plans to remake it in Hollywood so that the citizens of the USA (with whom we have a 'special relationship') can share it with us! The *plot* of the new film however will be referred to as the *story-line*, so that our ex-colonial cousins do not think it is something to do with a conspiracy.

To get back to the cogwheels, the idea was that the three cogwheels all turned round because they were inextricably linked with each other. Some of our colleagues set the date of the Revolution as the beginning of Cogwheel since this was an early attempt to imply that the drain sniffers were equal in status to hospital consultants and GPs and that this was the proverbial thin end of the wedge. Although the three cogs were initially all meant to represent doctors (i.e. hospital, general practitioner and community medical care[ii], it was only a few years later that the cogwheels actually became labelled. Now, in a sinister Orwellian manner it was the same three cogs, but they had become 'administration', 'medical' and 'nursing'. The authors think it noteworthy that the revisionists never thought to mention the patient!

There is an important legal concept known as res ipsa loquitur[22] which we will translate into English for the benefit of any Stasi (hospital administrator), who may even now still be reading this book: it means 'the thing speaks for itself'; the idea does not need any explanation – it is a self-evident fact. One such concept, which doctors have always taken for granted and never really thought needed explanation or debate, is the somewhat egocentric idea that they themselves are the most important members of the hospital team! The reader is reminded of the words of Albert Schweitzer, which appear in the prolegomenon. This notion, because it assumes superiority, is by definition patronising, but surely it is honest and no

---

[22]In a court case in Northern Ireland, involving an industrial dispute, the judge is said to have asked the plaintiff's barrister, 'Can the Court assume that your client is fully cognizant of the concept of res ipsa loquitur?' The defending barrister is reported to have looked over the top of his spectacles and replied, 'M'lud, the lads in the laundry talk of little else!'

less patronising than showing three interdigitated cogwheels, and implying the Stasi are as important as the medical and nursing staff, let alone the patient; (it is still the misguided belief of those supercilious, patronising doctors that the hospitals exist for the good of the patients). Cogwheel, however, was only the beginning. Within a few years, the Stasi themselves would come to look back on it with scorn. In the not too far distant future, they would no longer think of themselves as equal cogwheels, but, like the pigs in *Animal Farm*, sought total supremacy.

The Stasi themselves believe moreover that they have almost achieved superiority, although this is not the perception of the man in the street. People find it a shock when they arrive afresh in the present hospital system. The new Chairman of one Trust, on arriving at his new job, was very surprised to find that the consultants' offices were far smaller (and much less plush) than those for the Stasi. The reason why he was so surprised was that he had worked for the Police Federation before and had no real idea what went on in hospitals: he did of course have presupposed notions, but suddenly found that his presumption was completely wrong. He promised the consultants (whom he had on his arrival addressed as 'Sir'), that his first task would be to improve their office facilities. They smiled.

Sit Not Down in the Highest Room[23]

In the District General Hospital where one of the authors works, the size of the CEO's office was roughly three times the size of the senior consultant surgeon's office. He happened to mention this

---

[23]In Christ's parable of the Great Banquet, where everyone wants to sit at the top table, Jesus commends a genuinely humble spirit, not false modesty (St Luke, Ch 14 v 8).

fact to her secretary[24], who was very quick to point out defensively that the matriarch had to hold important meetings in this hallowed room. The secretary was not able, however, to explain why her own office (i.e. the secretary's)[25] was itself one and a half times as big. At this point your author forbore to point out the fact that the CEO and her minion had one office each. He had already got the impression that his having mentioned the fact that this 'royal suite' had wall-to-wall carpets, easy chairs and potted plants was considered not only unnecessarily inquisitive but also somewhat provocative.

On the subject of office paraphernalia, this is perhaps an appropriate moment to mention that the same hospital switchboard owned one – and only one – cell phone. It was not for the use of the Consultant in charge of Intensive Care or the Casualty Consultant. Perhaps our reader has already guessed who is accorded the privilege: the Stasi-On-Call. This does pose the interesting question of what does Stasi actually do when on call. One certainly wonders what life-threatening emergencies Stasi would be expected to deal with. Bed allocation, when one ward was full, was always done on a consultant-to-consultant basis. Whilst our readers are pondering this subject, they may rest assured that if they ever find out, they can ring her on her cell phone to confirm and she will be available at any time of day or night to respond to the life or death question (this might well be after she has rung up the appropriate consultant to find out what to say; they are after all called consultants).

It could be that the Stasi have considered the matter in depth

---

[24]He had to say something on being found in the CEO's office with a tape measure measuring the walls!

[25]Which your author had already measured before her intrusion.

and have concluded that senior doctors on call don't need a cell phone anyway as they should be required to remain on site and sleep at the hospital in the palatial accommodation provided, to deal with far less important calls (such as cardiac arrests, diabetic coma, haemorrhage, etc).

A delusion can be defined as a totally unfounded belief, which has a stronger hold on the mind than reality, so that demonstration of its falseness does not convince the deluded person. 'Delusions of Grandeur' used to be said to be a feature of the late (tertiary) form of syphilis (a disease which is now very rare). It is common practice for the Stasi to insist that their name appears on the bottom of all hospital writing paper[26]. This, of course, is not absolute proof of a grandiose delusional state (even less of tertiary syphilis), but is does say something about the arrogance of the perpetrator, who on arriving at a new hospital insists on the withdrawal of all the old stationery and then has nice new paper expensively printed (from NHS resources), each sheet bearing her or his own name.

This particular piece of egocentricity has other disadvantages in addition to extra printing costs. The Stasi have a notoriously short local shelf life, as they chop and change their jobs with great rapidity, so the writing paper's life is also short, incurring even greater cost. Your authors know of at least two consultants, and assume there must be many more throughout the country, who refuse to send out letters bearing the names of the Chairman and Chief Executive and so their over-worked secretaries have to spend unnecessary extra time with the paper guillotine cutting off the bottom inch of paper bearing the offending names. The authors

---

[26]The name of the headmistress of your author's daughters' school also appears on the bottom of the school writing paper.

nevertheless strongly recommend this simple procedure that prevents the names of, for example, an accountant and a retired Air Chief Marshall (who are not even remotely responsible[27] for the medical advice and opinion contained) being appended to a General Practitioner letter. It is further suggested that the strips of paper, which are cut off, are collected and put in an envelope like pasta, which is then sent to the Chief Executive with a compliments slip. In one hospital in the South West, this appeared to put an end to the extra printing.

Doctors' Titles and Their Origins

Not only has the trust of those whom the NHS serves been well nigh lost, but the trust of those who actually work for it has also been sorely tested. Cutbacks and closures are always widely reported, but more subtle changes often go unheeded. Doctors have even become worried about the title 'consultant'. This is not protected by law and there is nothing to stop others using it[28]. Physiotherapists, dieticians and nurses have, to the anger of many medical consultants, been adopting this title. In this, they are no different from the many financial consultants[29] and others who have latched onto the name. Yet, doctors have felt obliged to point out that use of the title 'consultant' by non-medically-qualified professionals not only confuses patients but also 'will eventually undermine standards in medicine'.[iii]

---

[27]'Power without responsibility,' was said by Rudyard Kipling to be, 'The prerogative of the harlot throughout the ages'.

[28]A 'sniffy' letter was published in the *BMA* News Review entitled 'We must be alert to "other consultants"' (March 1996, p10).

[29]When your authors were young men, they both remember financial consultants wearing gabardine raincoats knocking on their parents' back doors to collect premiums for the Prudential; in those days they were called 'insurance men'.

Patients also seem to be suffering from a new title. There is a definite move afoot to call them *Clients*! A point to note for the pedantic (or, considering the widespread use of such terms and the interest they create, the not-so-pedantic) is that:

- a 'Client' is in receipt of professional services, for which he pays[30];
- a 'Customer' is in receipt of trade or artisan services, for which he pays;
- an 'Applicant' is in receipt of professional services, for which he does not pay.

The misuse of correct English is usually the prerogative of the Stasi, but it must be said that some of one's psychiatric colleagues (should that have a capital P, or is that a Freudian slip in itself?) used to call their patients clients; believe it or not they now call them *Service Users*!

One of the authors wrote to the *Journal of the Royal Society of Medicine* (which was running a protracted discussion about what doctors should call their patients) pointing out the business of payment. It was also added that, in the current state of the NHS, a better term might be 'Supplicant' – who makes humble petition for things. The editor declined to publish his letter.

Have we always been so concerned with such matters? It seems that during the period 500 to 300 BC when all was flourishing in Ancient Greece, that nothing was written (or at least nothing has come down to us) on the question of medical etiquette[iv]. There are no references to etiquette in the earlier treatises of the Hippocratic collection either, but they do appear

---

[30]Prostitutes and Lawyers have 'Clients;' Doctors have 'Patients'.

later. This may be connected with the decline in the dignity of the medical profession.... As the status of medicine fell, less desirable characters became doctors. Those who cared for 'the art' (as it was always called), felt obliged to set down rules in writing. This is something to reflect on when another weighty and prescriptive tome from the GMC thuds onto the doormat.

Of course, right at the very beginning, the practice of the earliest doctors was one of naïve empiricism.[v] It was simply trial and error and a crude reliance on experience that showed the way to relieve pain and restore function. Herodotus tells of an ancient Babylonian custom of exposing the sick on highways where the pity and experience of passers-by were invoked.[vi] Some were healed and others died. It was only with time and experience that it became apparent which treatments were harmful and which were useful. The implication became that the dispenser of advice *knows*. Those who dispense advice had to have confidence in their knowledge and experience. Some anthropologists have identified 'primitive' patients who are prone to a deep despair and despondency (technically called thanatomania). For such people security lies only in belief in their healer's knowledge.[vii]

As time went by, the causes for disease were sought. Crude empiricism gave way to demonology. The primitive healer became a professional medicine man, privy to the animated world of disease and its cure. The art of healing has passed through four distinct phases[viii]. This started with the chief of a family in charge of the family's health (Patriarchal Phase). Then the healing art was usurped by the priesthood (Sacerdotal Phase). This reigned long in Ancient Egypt, flourished in Greece prior to Hippocrates, and reappeared in Europe during the Middle Ages. This was not very advantageous to surgery as the

THE HOSPITAL REVOLUTION

letting of blood and studies of anatomy by dissection were forbidden to priests. Midwifery also suffered as the sacred precincts of temples would have been profaned by birth or death. These subjects therefore grew up outside the established medical fraternity. Community medicine (had it existed) would probably have thrived in such settings though! This was followed by an Unlicensed Secular Phase and finally a Licensed or Organized Secular Phase in which medicine and surgery were combined outside the priesthood and its limitations.

The development of medicine in temples was helped by the fact that ancient peoples not only believed healing to be the gift of the gods, but that pestilence, disease and death were punishments from them. To regain the favour of the gods was to regain health. Hence, in its origin, healing was intimately connected with religion and mythology. Those who had been cured, perhaps by a neighbour or passer-by (see above) were required to have inscribed in the temples their disease and the method of its cure. From the mass of data, the priests formed a medical code. In this, medicine became the prerogative of the priesthood, who alone had access to the records and the necessary education to understand them. The temples became dispensaries in which advice was given and remedies administered.

We should consider specialization, which, according to Herodotus, achieved its zenith amongst the ancient Egyptians:

The medical profession is distributed among them (the Egyptians) in this way: each physician is for a single disease, and not for more. The whole land swarms with physicians: some are appointed for the eye, some for the head, some for

22

the teeth, others for the region of the belly, others again for unseen disease.

Herodotus ii 84

Throughout the nineteenth century in Britain, specialists who confined themselves to specific procedures were likely to be regarded as quacks. This is in complete contrast to nowadays[31] – something which not everybody approves of; as Niels Bohr said: 'An expert is someone who has made all the mistakes which can be made in a very narrow field.'

There was in fact a tripartite division of the medical profession up to the latter part of Victorian times according to the defining licences. These were the Physicians (controlled by the Royal College of Physicians), the Surgeons (controlled by their own colleges) and the Apothecaries under the control of the Worshipful Society of Apothecaries (London) and Apothecaries' Hall (Dublin). Only the physicians were entitled to the appellation 'doctor', something the surgeons continue to this day. This is a form of inverted snobbery, as the surgeons were stigmatized by their association with manual labour. But they were not as low as the apothecaries, who not only worked with their hands but were also associated with trade. A practitioner could only transfer allegiance by renouncing his

---

[31]There are those members of our profession who can become so wrapped up in their (very important) work that they become distanced from the realities of the rest of medical life – this is often to the detriment of the profession as a whole, and usually to the detriment of their own personal lives and relationships. Specialization breeds Tunnel Vision: We were shown a medical report written by an eminent otologist (some might say *the* most eminent otologist) regarding a post-operative facial paralysis. He considered this to be 'one of the most devastating injuries that could befall a patient'. The reaction of a midwife colleague was that he clearly had never witnessed a stillbirth or cot death; one can think of many other examples.

former calling. In reality, they all tended to work as general practitioners and were totally uncontrolled.[ix]

Certainly, not all surgeons made a living solely from surgery. Those practitioners who were already well established monopolised the hospitals. Consequently, it is not surprising that the response from younger aspiring specialists was to set up their own specialist hospitals. In so doing they could not only set themselves up in practice but also break the monopoly of the general hospitals[x].

The role of paramedical activities must also be considered. These were beginning to acquire a recognised place in the medical division of labour in the late nineteenth century. Massage had been newly legitimised as an auxiliary treatment in hospitals (the Society of Trained Massage being founded in 1894)[xi] and the discovery of X-rays allowed a new group of workers associated with this to develop[xii]. It was considered then, and still is, that by collaboration between members of a therapeutic and diagnostic team, a better result was obtained for the patient. The cynic might add, 'Until something goes wrong!' Such collaboration maintained a somewhat hierarchical structure. As a result of this partnership, management and administration grew in importance in order to ensure that the consumers' needs were met.... We thus see a change in authority, but not necessarily in responsibility. With the increasing specialization of medicine, medical authority began to pass from the expert coping single-handedly to institutions and groups of workers. Leadership became a necessary part of the repertoire of a consultant.

It is true that each decade has shown an increase in the number of medical practitioners and virtually every grade of hospital doctor. But the total amount of work to be done has also increased, if not *pari passu*.

This is slippery ground indeed. If we are to define something simply in terms of how good practitioners practise it, and then leave it up to those practitioners to set their own standards of what is good practice, then the unscrupulous will have a field day.

CHAPTER 2

MORALE

The Spoken Word above All

Both the authors hold a Queen's Commission and as such, in addition to being consultant surgeons have a second profession[1]. Although the Army has never really been particularly well known for teaching diplomacy skills[2], it does nonetheless allow one to acquire management and administrative ability. It certainly teaches leadership. During a quite acrimonious exchange of opinions with a female Stasi, one of your authors, who had

---

[1] On a purely philosophical note, here, it could be said that your authors had only one profession (i.e. the Army). Classically a professional person was one who professed as a calling one of the learned or liberal vocations, as opposed to a trade or business. This limited a gentleman's professions to the Church, the Law and the Army (physicians and more especially surgeons, who after all, were only glorified barbers, were tradesman – and even as late as the nineteenth century relegated to the tradesmen's entrance). Your authors do not wish to dwell on the profession open to 'ladies' in such a polite book as this; suffice it to say that it is not accountancy.

[2] But then diplomacy has never cured many patients.

formerly been the Commanding Officer of a 700-bedded Field Hospital, happened to point out to his adversary, in the most diplomatic manner, that he had run a bigger hospital than the one she was now in charge of and that he was more than confident that he could perform her job as well, if not better, than her, and assured her that she could not (nor was ever likely to be able to) even start to perform his job (specialised ear surgery). He never usually (for shame) mentioned the post-nominal qualifications he had obtained, whilst in the Army for management, but thought that this might now be an appropriate opportunity. After her initial dismay at learning of his management credentials, she stammeringly asked: 'Well, an Army hospital is not quite the same thing is it?'

The reverberations from dropping jaws were detected on MoD equipment miles away! With all the forbearance he could muster, he pointed out that it certainly was not. As Commanding Officer he had known all the names of all his officers, and most of his soldiers and quite often their spouse's and families' names. He had known and respected and looked after them; they had reciprocated. They would (at least he thought they would) have followed him anywhere. Most of all, he told her, the biggest difference of all, which the Field Hospital had, and she would never be able to muster, was *morale*.

Surely what is missing from the NHS today is morale. How can one hope to go forward with pessimism? Morale comes from leadership. Field Marshall Montgomery said:

Generals must see to it that their troops are imbued with infective optimism and that offensive eagerness which comes from physical well-being. Given this, and in the sure knowledge that they have a great and righteous cause, then must follow the will to persevere in battle in the face of all difficulties – and finally to conquer.[i]

Which great-thinking politician ever thought that doctors could ever be led by accountants? Once again we invoke the feelings of Lord Montgomery who maintained that men were 'the raw material of his trade:'[ii] they are certainly the raw material of the health service. It was essential for those men to know that someone cared for them. Monty knew that morale stemmed from leadership, and he himself was undoubtedly a great leader. He also knew that 'it is the spoken word above all which counts in the leadership of men'[iii]. He would jump on the bonnet of a jeep to give an impromptu address and stop to speak to men in a gun pit or by the roadside. They had no doubt whatsoever that he loved his men (in the nicest possible way) and had their best possible interests at heart. Compare this with the mealy-mouthed mousey accountants who cloister themselves among stacks of papers and are never seen beyond the confines of the Admin. Department[3].

Mind you, talking to the troops sometimes goes awry. Field Marshal Sir Douglas Haig evidently had always inspected his troops in silence, so one day it was suggested to him by one of his staff officers that it might be a good idea to stop and talk to one or two of the men. However, this only happened once. Haig stopped and asked one of the soldiers in the Yorks and Lancs Regiment:

'Where did you start this war, then, Private?'

The soldier looked bewildered and replied, 'I didn't start this war sir; I think it was the Kaiser.'

Evidently the Field Marshal did not realise the man was joking,

---

[3]Between 10 am and 2.30 pm, that is.

and never spoke to troops again. Most health service managers are not known for their humour, or come to that, their leadership.

For A Ha'p'orth Of Tar[4]

In the summer of 2000, the President of the Royal college of Surgeons of England said that 'frustration and despondency is at an alarming all time high'. Dr Philip Keep, a consultant anaesthetist in East Anglia, believes it has been killed by penny-pinching, and this is undoubtedly an important factor. He gives an eloquent example:

> Not too many years ago when an on-call surgeon had performed an emergency operation in the middle of the night, he and all the rest of the team – houseman, anaesthetist, scrub nurse, theatre technician, porter, and for that matter anyone who was around helping, would always be offered a free plate of bacon and eggs and cup of tea.

These were the days when that multi-disciplinary team[5]

> felt valued and cherished, and felt they were all in this thing together... a plate of free scrambled eggs at three in the morning bought fifty times its own value in ungrudgingly given effort.[iv]

When the Stasi were looking to save money, this was an immediate

---

[4]Evidently, one originally did not spoil the *ship* but the *sheep* for a halfpennyworth of tar! (Camdben W, 1614 *Remaines Concerning Britain*).

[5]The bureaucrats now make a (pathetic) point of trying to include themselves in multi-disciplinary teams.

soft target (and, of course, the Stasi are *never* in at 3 am). Free meals in the night were axed. What price goodwill? As night follows day, morale slips irretrievably away. One Stasi was actually heard to say, 'We're not running a Charity, you know.' Perhaps that was his basic error. Everyone knows that the NHS *is* a charity (an official public organisation for the relief of suffering). How many bacon sandwiches after all are equivalent to the price of an emergency operation? Laverne, the lovely uncomplaining plump West Indian who made the aforesaid bacon and eggs has been replaced by an automaton machine the size of an old red telephone kiosk, in which a carousel of uncooked meals revolve, alongside chocolate bars and bags of crisps, waiting for some unsuspecting night worker to lose a succession of one-pound coins in a fruitless attempt to activate the contained microwave oven.

It is certainly only a generation ago, when, on Christmas Day all the team would go together with their families to the hospital at lunchtime: there was never any question about it; it wasn't considered a duty (or for that matter a privilege) – they simply went because they had always gone. The boss of the firm would carve the ward turkey after everybody had done a festive ward round and exchanged seasonal greetings with the poor souls who through no fault of their own found themselves in a hospital bed on Christmas Day. After carving the turkey all the staff (doctors, nurses, cleaners and spouses)[6] would sit down with the patients and pull crackers and drink beer or wine which had been supplied by the consultants (the turkey dinner was always supplied free by the hospital).

Our readers will not be too surprised to learn that the spirit of Scrooge lives on in the Stasi who have put a stop to all this

---

[6]Even in those days, the Stasi never came.

unnecessary largesse. However, it would be grossly unfair if the munificence of the Birmingham hospitals were not mentioned. Clearly the accusation of Scroogian humbug cannot be justifiably levelled at them. The East Birmingham Trust announced with a degree of pride prior to Christmas 1997 that during the season of goodwill they would provide doctors who were on duty on Christmas Day with free *sandwiches*. Readers will surely agree that such bounty should not pass unrecognised, and perhaps also concur that those who remained on duty were ungracious to turn down their free ham sandwiches to go and eat more festive seasonal fare in their élitist doctors' mess (which was later closed down).

Food in Resident Doctors' Messes always used to be free before the Revolution. In some hospitals there even used to be free beer. We can both remember with affection the free Boddington's beer which used to be supplied to the Manchester Ear Hospital for the staff (presumably because one of the Boddington family had good reason to be grateful to that institution which was quite close to the Strangeways Brewery). Those days are sadly over: there is no longer free food or beer for staff who work unsocial hours (and the Manchester Ear Hospital has been closed down. Come to think of it, Boddington's Beer has never tasted quite as good to us since the brewery was computerised in April 1997). Even in the large teaching hospital messes, on-call doctors no longer get the midnight feasts when they are called out.

Dr Keep points out that it is the NHS employees themselves who are continually being asked to make such sacrifices for the good of patient care. He compares it to charging soldiers for every round of ammunition they shoot, and points out that before the Revolution, the old *undermanaged* NHS did have one great commodity – morale. It used to be the only working model of a truly effective communist system. It had the absolute goodwill of its workforce who used to hold old-fashioned élitist values and the now out-dated ethic about the importance of the patient. It was a case of: 'From each according to his ability; unto each according to his need[7] and it was astounding how great people's ability was, and how small their needs were.'

Before the Revolution, people felt valued and had self-esteem; they felt they were all part of a team and they all pulled together. In those distant days even the Hospital Secretary (amazingly) was considered as part of that team. Although there was undoubtedly some wastefulness and profligacy in some areas, the NHS workers never got many perks. They never got free company cars, share options, profit-sharing bonus schemes or trips abroad – though having said this, some Trusts evidently have a 10% discount with local undertakers. Nonetheless they gave of their best and there was a certain pride in working for the fuddle-brained NHS.

There was above all *goodwill*.

And they have killed it!

Above and Beyond the Call?

Not too many years ago, not a thousand miles away from the Edgbaston cricket ground, a dear friend of ours, called Ivor, was appointed consultant ENT surgeon. On his arrival he found that he had inherited a two-and-a-half year waiting list for tonsillectomies

---

[7]This is usually attributed to Karl Marx in his famous *Criticism of the Gotha Programme* of 1875. In fact the old revolutionary had plagiarised it from the anarchist, Michael Bakunin, who had used these precise words five years previously (1870) in a declaration of forty-seven anarchists on trial after the failure of their uprising in Lyon – Morrison Davidson J. *The Old Order and the New*, 1890.

and nose jobs[8]. As a gesture of goodwill, he promised that he and his team would operate throughout the night for a number of weeks until he had got rid of what he considered to be *his* waiting list. We emphasise the word *his* because in the pre-Revolution days, a consultant considered the amount of time NHS patients under his nominal care had to wait, to constitute *his* personal NHS waiting list. Nowadays, sadly we have moved away from this paternalistic attitude and have been ordered to consider this to be the Trust's waiting list.

Ivor, with the cooperation of the theatre staff and even the anaesthetists (!) worked through the night in 1980 to cut down the waiting list for his patients, because he had an old-fashioned paternalistic attitude towards them and actually cared about their welfare. He had an obsolete sense of duty and responsibility and actually wanted to provide a high quality service.

He did not ask for money for this service.

The hospital held his goodwill; he felt valued – even cherished – and gave his time unquestioningly. Sadly this is no longer the case. If a surgeon nowadays is asked to do an extra list, he is offered a fee! It is usually derisory, and as a result the operating list is delegated to a junior (in the same way as a lump of sugar is offered to a pet horse). The accountants have moved in and are trying to run the NHS like a supermarket. Now when a waiting list is going well beyond the levels of the Patient Charter the Stasi undertake what they call a Waiting List Initiative. This is an extra list that would not normally be undertaken, and performed at a

---

[8]In 1982 a patient from Birmingham emigrated to Ilfracombe and asked the North Devon ENT surgeon if he could be put one year up the North Devon waiting list for his 'nose job' (septoplasty) owing to the fact that he had already been waiting a year in Brum. The surgeon laughed and told him he wished he could, and then it would already have been done three months ago!

time when no list would normally be done. The managers try to arrange them during the working day. That way they can cut back on any extra money to be doled out.

Of course, many of the Stasi who have arranged this initiative list are on an efficiency bonus system. They have a large financial incentive to speed things through before the end of the financial year. There is no altruism.

Whereas before the Revolution, the doctors would work ungrudgingly and unquestioningly and seek for no reward, now when asked if they will do an initiative, the first question which is asked is sadly, 'How much money will I get?' In this way we have prostituted ourselves. Ten years ago we would never have dreamed of asking for money for the privilege of cutting down what were then *our* waiting lists. Sir Lancelot Spratt would never have dreamed of asking for remuneration for doing extra NHS operating lists.

Sister Susan would never have dreamed of taking the morning off sick to go to the doctor with backache before the Revolution. She would have gone to work and suffered during the day and gone to the evening surgery after work. She had never taken a day off sick for thirty-three years since being a student nurse and had become a sister at a well-known children's hospital in the North of England. Before the Revolution, she had loved her work and enjoyed every minute at the hospital. Indeed her husband and children had grumbled about her excessive commitment. She was a professional nurse of the old school and dedicated to her profession and her patients. Recently however, she had seen changes take place in the out-patients department which sickened her. A Stasi younger than Sister Susan had been appointed as Outpatient Manager. She was not as well-qualified and had nowhere near as much experience. She had certain *aims*. The main goal was to remove nurses from outpatients' clinics. Before when one attended the clinic, one could expect to be ushered in by a qualified nurse who would have experience of dealing with sick people, help them to undress, provide moral and physical support and explain details to the patient. This was the least they would do. In certain instances they would undertake treatments, apply dressings, remove stitches, etc. Each doctor would be allocated a nurse. No longer. 'It is not cost effective.' In some hospitals, they don't even get a nursing auxiliary. It is interesting to note that, whereas outpatient clinics have become busier with more investigations and procedures being done on an outpatient basis, the staff are fewer and less skilled (management-speak is 'deskilling the job'). In contrast, on the other side of the house, wages clerks are to be found dressed up as financial managers with personal assistants, etc.

Sister Susan had even seen the telephones removed from consultants' consulting rooms because time spent on the telephone was detracting from outpatient clinic resources. She herself had blamed the complacent doctors for allowing these changes to take place. They would never have got away with it with the old professor (Sir Lancelot would never have stood for it!). Now the school-leaver Outpatient Manager had turned her attention to Sister Susan and was quickly coming to the conclusion that she was supernumerary. In order to release more money to pay the salaries of newly appointed Stasi, cuts had necessarily been made, and those cuts had hit the nurses. Now there was the bare minimum of trained nurses to keep the wards running and the plan was clear that Sister Susan's nursing skills could be more effectively utilised upstairs on the wards.

She certainly had backache that morning, but whereas in the past she would have soldiered on, now her commitment had been eroded. Whereas before the old professor would have supported her and respected her commitment, the new manager made sure that she didn't have much contact with the young professor. In short, whereas before, Susan had felt *valued*, she was no longer too sure. After all, they had a long-term plan to shift her upstairs onto the wards (where she would have to work different shifts which wouldn't fit in with her children's school times, and so she would probably leave). The more Susan thought about it, the more sure she became aware that she wasn't valued any more, and so the more convinced she became that she would behave like everybody else and go to see her GP. She would no longer continue to behave like a dutiful professional nurse who she knew was different after all, certainly to the financially driven Stasi who know nothing about loyalty to patients and to colleagues.

Sister Susan no longer felt valued.

This is now a commonplace in the new Health Service.

The malaise is not confined simply to the wards and clinics. Many young secretaries do sterling work and they are certainly being utterly demoralised by the new regime. They often have hard-earned qualifications in shorthand and typing, and some have the prestigious diploma of medical secretaries. It must be particularly galling when dictatorial women with no qualifications (who cannot do anything properly, let alone type) and who have never been a secretary – never worked *in the field* as it were – hire and fire them and determine their conditions of service.

Respect is a brittle and intangible quality, which has to be earned; it does not come automatically with rank and status. All Chief Constables in this country started their professional life as policemen on the beat, and the bobbies who are still on the beat know that fact and respect their chief for it. Admirals all started as midshipmen. Captains of merchant ships have all worked on the deck before rising through the ranks to the bridge. So it is (and should be) with any proper hierarchical system. A fireman will respect his Fire Chief if he knows that his boss too has been through it all himself and climbed ladders and broken down doors of burning buildings. The reverse is also true: he would have scant respect for a new Fire Chief who was an accountant and who had never worn breathing apparatus or fought to control a gushing hose. Perhaps respect is not something that is needed or sought. A friend of the authors draws our attention to a sentence he read in a management article: 'Management is a skill unrelated to knowledge of that which is managed.'

This might explain a lot.

The most commonly quoted reason for poor industrial relations is poor communication. How can the Stasi hope to understand the secretaries' plight when they have not only never done any secretarial work, but usually have never set foot in a hospital office outside their own? Ask any of the medical secretaries if they have ever seen their admin. bosses and more than 90 per cent will say they have not. So much for the greatest factor in morale being the spoken word: it becomes rather difficult to communicate orally if you have never met! It would appear that things are not quite as bad for nurses. A staff nurse recently told one of us that in the hospital in which she now worked (and the previous two), she had never actually met the Director of Nursing (our readers have probably guessed that this is newspeak for 'Matron'). She went on, however, to say that the only time she had ever met one was on the day she qualified, when she actually shook hands with one, who said the single word 'Congratulations!' to her. No oral communication has taken place between them since, however.

In the fourteenth century, the practice of bloodletting was very popular as it was thought to get rid of evil humours in the blood by simply letting them out. The actual *timing* of when the vein was opened was based on astrological considerations. Surprisingly, we can assure you that the best time to have your appendix out (on the NHS) is probably still at the cusp of the signs of Cancer and Leo. The reason for this, however, is nothing at all to do with the stars. It is because the housemen (who would almost certainly perform the operation) work on an annual rotation, which starts every year on 1st August after graduating from medical school in July. By the end of January they will have been a houseman for six months and change at this time from medicine to surgery or vice versa. It follows, therefore, that by the end of the following July (apparently the cusp of Cancer and Leo) they are quite experienced in both arts of medicine and surgery, and therefore more likely to be more competent at taking your appendix out than the houseman during August, who has only just left Medical School and therefore has hardly any experience.

During July 1997, one of us was at a very pleasant party at the Doctors' Mess of a district general hospital, which was the housemen's farewell bash. Talking to some of the junior doctors who had been working there for at least six and in most cases nearly twelve months, the topic of conversation came round, perhaps inevitably, to the Stasi. The author was quite surprised to find out that the young houseman who was talking had no idea of the name of the chief executive (or the chairman) of the Trust in which he had worked for a year. On questioning others in the immediate vicinity, it became apparent that six out of the seven asked did not know the name of the CEO, and none of them had ever met her, spoken to her or heard her voice. So much for Monty's maxim about the spoken word. No wonder morale is low.

Three of the seven housemen in question also said that they intended to emigrate. The CEO may not be directly responsible for the 'brain drain', but she is certainly wholly and personally responsible for the low morale in that hospital. It is a disgrace that she did not know the housemen. The truth is that the Stasi hardly ever venture beyond their own corridors of power. The administration department in most hospitals is usually the only area where the offices are large and have carpets[9]. Because the Stasi never venture out of the admin. department, they remain unknown. In two hospitals known to us, at different ends of the country, the Director of Nursing has never been seen on the wards. Perhaps she considers it beneath her dignity. Suffice to say she is not respected by the nurses (despite the fact that she does hold a nursing qualification!). She is quite often *away* at an important meeting and is never seen outside *office hours* even in the admin. block.

Compare this with the good old Matron. She would know all her nurses' names and talk to them all on a regular basis. She would visit all the wards and talk to all the ward sisters (and also the patients). If any of the nurses had any problems they would take them to the Matron and she would listen and sort them out. Matrons were not always *loved* by their staff, but they were always *respected*, and with that respect came stability and a feeling of trust that all was in good hands. This solid reliability and trust[10] strengthened the morale, which was a great feature of the old hospital system.

The Postgraduate Secretary is a very important post in hospitals, being concerned with the organisation of most of the

---

[9]The reason once actually stated for the carpets (and the authors emphasise to the dear reader who, although not naïve, is probably kinder and more trusting than the average cove, that this is *not* a joke) is that the carpets damped down the noise (this Stasi was well-informed) and therefore the carpets prevented eavesdropping at job interviews!

[10]It is important here that the word trust does not have a capital 't'.

continuing teaching and education for the doctors (something we had learnt to call CME – Continued Medical Education – before a new abbreviation, CPD – Continued Professional Development – was thrust upon us). Doctors have always had a good record of updating their knowledge and skills, and have always continued to read professional journals and go on courses to keep them aware of the ever-accelerating progress which medical sciences continue to make. The Post-Graduate Centre Secretary has been an important coordinator in this work, liaising between lecturers and doctors and the pharmaceutical industry as well as makers of surgical instruments and also the library. All large hospitals have a Post-Graduate Medical Centre, and at an important one in Wessex[11] the Senior Secretary recently, after providing an excellent service for over thirty years, retired. The Authority decided not to replace her: it would cost too much money. They would muddle through with an audio typist. Some (a very limited number) of doctors made a very loud mutter, but didn't really put up any sort of confrontational offensive against the Director of Personnel (or 'Personal' as it was often mistakenly written), who evidently earned £n p.a. (where n is a very large number) and did not even have any A-levels. It was not that the doctors were gutless, or that they were ostriches. It was really because they weren't motivated enough: they didn't care enough for the woman who had done sterling service for them for so many years. And so she retired and was not replaced. The girl who got her job was to earn a salary less than the retiring secretary's assistant!

What did that do for the morale of the Post-Graduate Department? The lady retiring was terribly depressed and felt under-valued – as though all the years she had put in of hard work had been not only

---

[11] That is Thomas Hardy's Wessex rather than any other.

unappreciated but not even needed. Her 'replacement' was working in an office nominally in charge of a secretary who was earning more money. The new Post-Graduate Secretary came to resent her subordinate intensely. In the acrimony that followed the assistant left for another post in the same hospital, despite many years (considerably more than her new 'boss') of experience of the workings of her old office. What a masterpiece of mismanagement! The Stasi who had perpetrated it left shortly afterwards; he was promoted to Director of Human Resources (despite his not having an A-level) at an even larger hospital.

One supposes the replacement should have thought him or herself lucky that at least she had got a full contract. One penny-pinching method is not to appoint definitive replacements when somebody retires or leaves, but to put in a locum and to make double sure that that locum doesn't work there for more than two years. That way they can be dismissed and the Trust will not have to pay her any redundancy payments.

The Patients' Charter is cited as another cause for discontent. A Doctor and Nurses' Charter would have been a more sensible move, to protect a once well-motivated and irreplaceable workforce from increasingly ill-mannered, demanding and litigious patients as well as 'the enemy within', by which is meant the dark forces that are unable to discern the difference between practising the healing arts and selling a tin of paint. Dr John Grange, a microbiologist at London's Imperial College School of Medicine, considers the parsimonious attitude of the Stasi as just one of the causes in the vicious downward spiral of morale in hospital workers.[v] (In this book, the term 'hospital workers' is used to apply to those employees other than managers and administrators). Grange considers the major factor to be lack of communication with administration; he says that instead of meaningful dialogue:

We are tossed platitudes, ineptitudes, soundbites and claptrap because the underlying philosophy of health care provision is no longer based on rational and enlightened thinking, but on a dogmatic anti-intellectual and fundamentalist belief system. This demands that dissidents are, metaphorically, burned at the stake. As a result, staff are treated badly, morale declines, quality of work declines, patients feel ill-treated, complaints and litigation increase, costs rise and penny-pinching grows.

In the same way as the old Soviet totalitarian regime would brand dissidents as insane (after all they just had to be made to agree with the *system*) then condemn them to a lunatic asylum somewhere in Siberia, this is going on in the present NHS. Because he was not toeing the line, a consultant pathologist was asked by his Trust to see a psychiatrist. No mental health problem was found but the consultant was nonetheless frogmarched off the premises: there was no evidence of clinical incompetence whatsoever, but the pathologist was hounded by his Trust and eventually retired because of his bitterness at the vindictive behaviour towards him.[vi]

Trust and Confidence

One of the authors found himself in a very similar situation. He had not been accused of any clinical misdemeanour whatsoever, but was asked to attend a formal interview. This began with the CEO reiterating the fact that he was not being arraigned on a clinical matter. In fact, the CEO started off by telling him that she had every 'trust and confidence'[12] in him as a surgeon. Being a firm believer in

---

[12]The lady Chief Executive at first told him 'every trust and *confidentiality*'. She was quickly corrected by the Manager of Human Resources (personnel officer). We have found that Chief Executives have a poor command of English.

the *Timeo Danaos et dona ferentes*[13] principle, this put the author (who has been taught to be cautious) on his guard. There was also something about the way the woman seemed to stress the two words *trust* and *confidence*, almost hissing them. She had always reminded him of a reptile, but now her emotionless eyes and cold-looking skin put him particularly in mind of a female version of the serpent in the Garden of Eden! Whilst he was musing on this similarity, he heard her voice asking him for a similar affirmation of his trust and confidence in the senior management in the Trust administration! Luckily he was so taken aback that he did not immediately reply with the knee-jerk reaction he would not even trust her to take his dog for a walk. The author had also luckily had the foresight to take along a 'prisoner's friend' to this enforced confrontation who quickly intervened with a whispered warning that trusts had recently been getting rid of trouble-makers and whistleblowers by the 'lack of mutual trust and confidence' ploy. This *mutual* business was evidently why she had initially professed her undying confidence in his surgical dexterity.

'I can assure you, madam that I am very sure that I have a similar trust and confidence in you to that which you repose in me.'

Clearly infuriated that her spiteful plan was not going to work, she told him that this answer was not satisfactory and she must insist on another. Of course, none was forthcoming and a few seconds afterwards the interview was terminated when he decided that enough was enough, and politely excused himself to go and get another bacon sandwich from the hospital canteen[14].

---

[13]'Beware of Greeks bearing gifts' – Virgil Aeneid 2,49. A more modern writer, Tennessee Williams, held in *Camino Real* that, 'We have to distrust each other – it is our only defense against betrayal'.

[14]One has to grudgingly admit that the food during the day in hospital canteens seems to have improved following privatization. There was a period during the eighties when bacon was never used in the hospital, because the Stasi feared it might be stolen by the staff.

For Stasi to summon a consultant surgeon to a meeting in this manner is preposterous impudence in itself. She had, however, put her cold reptilian finger on it with unerring accuracy regarding trust and confidence. Why have things reached this level of lack of confidence and the lowest morale since the inception of the NHS?

Whistleblowers

The only 'crime' the author had committed, and which prompted this 'conversation', was speaking his mind. Let us for a moment look back at the pledge of Aneurin Bevan, who (for the benefit of any Stasi who are so thick-skinned as to still be reading this book, was a very well-meaning Welsh Labour M.P.[15] who started the National Health Service in 1948. Bevan promised all workers in the new NHS:

> You will be fully free to conduct agitation and vote against the Ministry of Health at any time you care. There will be no limitation at all upon the civil liberties of the persons working in the NHS.

More recently, however, owing to the fact that the Stasi are experiencing difficulty in controlling (and sometimes 'gagging') intellectually superior doctors[16] in their employ, the Rt Hon Mrs

---

[15] Is 'Welsh Labour M.P.' a tautology cf. 'dour Scotsman'? Would it not convey exactly the same meaning with economy of words to say 'Welsh M.P.' and 'Scotsman'? John Braine was thinking along similar lines when he described one of his characters as 'The meanest man in Yorkshire – which meant the meanest man in the world'. We are both from Yorkshire, and consider more correct adjectives would be careful, or frugal, rather than 'mean'.

[16] Another tautology?

Virginia Bottomley[17] clearly abrogated Nye Bevan's pledge as it applied to herself. She said:

> Any disclosure to the media of a matter which is relevant to the employee's work and responsibilities, without the consent of the employer might be seen by the employer as damaging the relationship of mutual trust and would therefore represent a potentially serious breach of contract.

The essence of this whole procedure was that of duty and loyalty[18]. It was evidently worrying to doctors in 1948. Some misguided critics would have you believe that the doctors' foremost anxieties about the forthcoming NHS were concerned with money. We are willing to admit that pecuniary interests did certainly give rise to some worry, but there were other much more fundamental concerns. The Medical and Dental Defence Union of Scotland published a book to commemorate the setting up of the NHS[vii] and on the fourth page drew attention to an editorial written in the *British Medical Journal* December 1947, some seven months beforehand:

> State medical service is something to which the medical profession has always been resolutely opposed, because it

---

[17](Tory) Secretary of State for Health.

[18]It should be noted that the origin of the rule that consultants should live within a specified distance of their hospital has nothing to do with availability for emergencies. When one considers how in the past doctors were called to an emergency (often by a porter wandering around the resident accommodation), this of course makes sense. The real reason was to imbue loyalty to the area. It was considered that by having senior members of staff in (relatively) close proximity, the status of the hospital would be enhanced and camaraderie fostered.

believes that the restrictions and frustrations of a State service geared to a top-heavy administrative machine would prevent that intellectual freedom which is so essential to medicine as a science and an art.

Those familiar with State enterprises were not surprised to read on page 15 an example of how this was manifesting itself:

> The work which eventually led to the development of Magnetic Resonance Imaging (MRI) was done by Professor Mallard in the early 1960s. In March 1974 his team managed to obtain an image of a whole mouse. A race began between six teams – four in the UK and two in the USA; a year was spent in obtaining a grant of £30,000 from the Medical Research Council... Multinational companies saw the potential and a prototype developed by General Electric of New York became available during 1982/3. By 1985 there were hundreds of imagers in use in the USA, Germany and Japan. In the UK, where it had been developed, there were barely ten!

The main fears of the profession, however, were with the more fundamental concern of the absolute nature of a doctor's commitment to an individual patient, without the interposition of a third party, be it the state or an insurance company – or any other individual or agency. Medicine is a profession, which like the Church or the Law marches to a different drum. Whenever doctors are face to face with a sick patient, duty, ethics and honour demand that no constraint be placed on them by an employer, government, or anyone else. They must do the best that can be done – *even to the extent that it is to the doctor's own detriment.*[viii]

The Stasi seem unable to even start to understand this concept at all. They think that the doctor's loyalty should be to his employer (a bit like the Japanese show to Mitsubishi or Toyota). They really have no idea at all that doctors have a very strange loyalty (which is peculiar to medicine) and it is directed primarily to their ill patients. What Mrs Bottomley did not understand is that the doctor does not really care two hoots about his employers and not a lot more for his colleagues[19] (by which we mean other doctors), but will go through hell and high water for his or her sick patient. The idea that his first duty should be to some intangible Trust, run by a group of low-grade, low-intelligence, incompetent accountants (who have probably never even seen a bed-pan[20]) is anathema. The first duty always has been to the poorly patient. And if it means speaking out to get what that suffering patient needs, then so be it. The employer is totally inconsequential. If the Stasi do not like it, it doesn't matter at all. That Mrs Bottomley should start to talk about 'serious breaches of contract' shows just how far out of the frame she was. And it underlines just how inappropriate it is to have medically unqualified persons in charge of the Health Service.

The Nolan Report of 1995[ix] ostensibly encouraged whistle-blowing (and coined the term). Later in the same year

---

[19] A consultant surgeon in Manchester whose hobby was stock breeding always used to maintain vociferously, 'I much prefer my cattle to my colleagues'.

[20] It might be considered that this deficit has no importance whatsoever. As has been said, 'The experience of marriage and parenthood is good fuel to any writer. Though we should note that few have written better about marriage and children than Jane Austen. The likes of Jane Austin are few and far between – she was a rare, special talent. The counter-argument might be that it is not important to have first hand experience because the talented person will not need to personally experience something in order to have insight.' The authors agree – let the reader by all means give the Stasi this leeway. But the authors would caution the reader – not all the Stasi are talented!

Whistleblowing in the Health Service[x] added its support and the following year the *BMA News Review* reported the overwhelming wave of magnanimity which was overtaking the NHS: eighty-three out of the 120 doctors who had been suspended over the past ten years had been re-instated! The Nolan Proposal, however, was far from being universally implemented, particularly in Trusts in Trent, North West Thames and West Midlands regions, and *Stalinism in the Health Service* (a term used in the *British Medical Journal* in December 1994)[xi] continued to be practised. The Stalinist Trusts chose to interpret the term 'whistleblowing' in a highly specific manner: indeed they appeared to welcome the practice insofar as it only ever applied to a doctor blowing the whistle on one of his colleagues (the so-called 'shop a doc' principle) but it should certainly never be used to criticise an authority!

One of the authors was threatened with disciplinary action in 1997 for what he considered was merely an exercise of his basic freedom of speech, and principally because of this, he wrote to Frank Dobson[21] to clarify whether his first duty was to his sick patients or to the Trust; would they be honouring Nye Bevan's pledge and would he still be free to 'conduct agitation... at any time.' The answer was somewhat guarded: 'On the question of a doctor's first duty, I am unequivocal – it is to the patients. However, a doctor has a duty to act reasonably towards his employer.'[xii] He added that he had written to the CEO telling her to lay off your poor author. Although this is not the 'unequivocal'

---

[21]A fact not generally known about this Minister of Health but which has been confided to your authors by two disenchanted London cabbies is that, on entering a black London taxi, he always pulls down the dickie seat and sits with his back to the engine (he is the son of a railwayman), even if he is alone. To our knowledge, this fact does not appear in any other book!

support as stated, this represents a change in attitude, which should be welcomed.

Should we not be trying to understand (and maybe even supporting) such 'whistleblowers'? They may not always be right, but it is a dangerous assumption that they are necessarily wrong. As Albert Einstein said: 'Few people are capable of expressing with equanimity opinions which differ from the prejudices of their social environment; most people are incapable of forming such opinions.'[xiii] Is it to be taken as read that freedom of speech is going to be compromised to this extent? Even the British Medical Association, which one would hope would be concerned to protect such freedoms, reports that these are not simply the mutterings of one errant politician, yet acknowledges that: 'The doctor's individual clinical freedom is no longer free-standing, it is an authority delegated by one's peers and embodied in a corporate clinical responsibility[xiv].

The first bit doesn't sound too bad, so long as one is quite clear about who constitutes one's 'peers'. The reader will be learning about the experiences of one of the authors in this matter shortly. Clinical freedom rarely flourishes in a vacuum and as a profession we are bound by our own professional rules and the regulations which come with being a member of a profession. But so much of what we do is inspected, quantified and contracted for by those who know nothing of our values – and probably care not a jot for them anyway. Or is that too cynical? The reader must decide after reading further. We contend that doctors speak up for what is right – otherwise we would not be doing our job. These sentiments were echoed at a day symposium 'NHS Day at the Royal Society of Medicine' held 8 July 1998, when Averil Mansfield spoke on Hospital Practice:[xv]

We are intelligent and at times voluble professionals and no one should feel surprise or regret that hospital doctors may want to express concerns about problems and deficiencies in that service from our viewpoint. Most of us do see it from a wider, indeed, international perspective but within that context will continue to be aware of the more parochial problems and try with all our might to address those concerns. *It simply indicates how much we care.*

Holier (More Politically Correct) Than Thou[22]

It has been said of your authors that we used to be cynical. This is no longer the case. Now we are bitter and twisted! However, a certain degree of cynicism should be brought to bear when dealing with the ever increasing phenomenon of 'reporting one's colleagues'. These tend not to be for clinical matters but the 'holier than thou' attitude of the busybody who feels obligated to seek out acts of racism and sexism, etc, usually where there is no case to answer. Presumably they are 'acting of behalf of those weaker and unable to speak for themselves' – which itself might well be construed as a racist or sexist act.

Is this pure altruism? We think that often this is not the case at all. The 'whistleblower' (who often has no real idea of what is going on, what has been said or done, etc) wades in with the self righteous manner of the bigot who knows what is what and what is right. They get a warm glowing feeling for 'having done the right thing', get asked to make statements, attend a meeting and

---

[22]'Holier than thou' is taken from the Old Testament (Isaiah, 65, v.5): 'Stand by thyself, come not near to me for I am holier than thou'. According to Biblical scholars, the odious PC misuse of words did not raise its ugly head until about 2,800 years afterwards.

feel important. Often the 'perpetrator' and 'victim' are completely bemused by the whole affair.

That is not to say that there are not acts of sexism, racism and the like which do go on and which should be deplored. The problem is that these days it is very easy to make an accusation and very difficult to defend oneself. The unscrupulous can easily use this to 'get back' at someone, or defend or improve their own position. A 'victim' of some slight can easily put in a report 'make an official complaint' which of course has to be investigated. Mud sticks, even when the 'perpetrator' is fully exonerated – often after a lengthy and worrying period of time. The complainant has by then established under what difficult circumstances they have had to work 'as one of the few or the only woman, ethnic minority, Blue Whale, Yorkshireman, etc. working in this department'. Clearly being the subject of bullying or acts of discrimination they should be given special treatment, advancement, not judged so harshly at their annual review. Perhaps we should be grateful for small mercies – unlike in the former Soviet Union or East Germany, at least the complaints are made openly rather than anonymously and the accused knows what is being said against him. Or does he? Perhaps we are being paranoid. But are we being paranoid enough?

Morale is essential to the health and wellbeing of any large organisation or body of people and morale in the health service started the millennium at an all-time low. The existence of vast armies of unnecessary Stasi making incompetent and meddlesome changes is one of the leading causes for this decline of what used to be a very happy system; most 'old hands' agree that the old NHS hospitals were satisfying places to work in, but in a variety of ways and not always for financial expediency. So-called managers have destroyed all the goodwill which used to exist. Your authors, two surgeons, would not wish to cause unnecessary alarm and despondency[23], but even they, usually so cheerful and light-hearted, cannot fail to admit to a profound sense of unease at the present low spirits they see all around them.

Sadly, they are not alone.

Last summer, they chanced to meet a dear friend in London on his way home from his annual family holiday. He is an experienced, respected and talented surgeon, at the peak of his career at a well-known teaching hospital. He told them that he had loved surgery since being a medical student thirty-five years ago, and had hitherto always looked forward to returning to work after a (well-earned) holiday. This year, however, he had felt differently. This was the first time in his long career that he had not looked forward to going back to work. The Stasi had got even to him and undermined his morale. He also said that until recently he had always intended to press on until he was sixty-five years old[24], but he would now 'get out' as soon as he could.

What a lamentable thing, but he is certainly not an isolated case.

A Veritable Slough of Despond[25]

The cumulative problems in working for the NHS is causing vast numbers of personnel to leave. In fact, if the NHS *was* a

---

[23]Behaviour likely to cause undue alarm and despondency was a Civil Offence during the Last War.

[24]This is despite the 'fact' quoted by many surgeons that if they retire at sixty, their life expectancy is more than twice that if they retire at sixty-five!

[25]This is borrowed from Bunyan's *Pilgrim's Progress* (1678) Author's Apology, Part 1, in which it is a deep bog Christian has to cross in order to reach the Wicket Gate. Help came to Christian in the shape of neighbour, Pliable, who accompanied Christian through the Slough of Despond.

commercially-run company as the Stasi would love us to believe, then such a loss would never be tolerated. It is only because the universities and training colleges (i.e. the taxpayer) foot so much of the training costs and they do not show up on the NHS balance sheet that the situation is allowed to continue.

Professor Domhnall MacAuley[26], a GP in West Belfast and Professor of Primary Healthcare Research (that word again!) at the University of Ulster, told a meeting of GPs that a few years ago they had been the keenest and cleverest of university graduates. If that is the case, and your authors contend that it probably is the case, then why are so many not coping, leaving, or even committing suicide?

What has the health service done to batter these doctors?

Addressing the Permanent Secretary at the Department, he said that the profession and the Health Department had to work together.[xvi] Our readers will no doubt by this stage realise that of all the things to do, this is probably least likely to help. It follows the same sort of thinking that if there is a problem then it might be solved by designing a new form or convening a committee. It is the authors' experience that this is hardly ever the case – things only get worse (but a lot more pen-pushers become employed).

Why do people leave medicine? Surveys by the British Medical Association may well produce dire predictions of those 'planning to take early retirement', or whatever. But one has to be aware of the nature of the question posed. Few people admit to being satisfied, and if a political point is to be made, then the threat of leaving the profession may be used as a lever. In contrast to this, Louis Appleby in his wonderful book *A Medical Tour through the whole Island of Great Britain*[xvii] recounts interviewing a fisherman.

---

[26]The authors have not made this name up.

He had undertaken this dangerous job all his working life – a total of thirty years, though there had been a gap during this time of two years when he had given it up. The reason? – he didn't like it.

It may be that medical students are leaving for the very same reason, but when one considers the lengths that people go to get into medical school, it seems strange that so soon after achieving this end so many should give up. In a study published in *Health Trends*[xviii] it was reported that 'the overall dropout rate from the combined London schools 1984–87 compared favourably with other UK medical schools.' So far, so good! We authors were staggered to read that the figures were from 7.2 to 11.2 per cent!

Something seems very wrong when about a tenth of the country's potential doctors give up before they have even started. The memory can play strange tricks but such a wastage rate never seemed to occur when we were undergraduates – and in those days there were many more opportunities to obtain alternative employment.

Another thing which has changed since those halcyon days is the number of overseas graduates in British Medical Schools. Britain has always had a good track record of looking after her former colonial subjects and indeed when JRY was dissecting cadavers in 1965, he not only learned human anatomy but also acquired a certain facility in Swahili! There have always been foreign students in our medical schools but Jim Johnson, chairman of the BMA's Consultants' Committee reported that only 38 per cent of the 4,970 doctors who qualified in 1997 were British-born.

With the dwindling number of trainees and the increasing number of early retirements, things are heading towards disaster. In June 1998 the British Medical Association announced the grim fact that the crisis is at present so great that: 'They have got to do something about this urgently, because if they don't the NHS is going to run out of doctors early in the new millennium.' The same month, *The Times* said that: '1,000 more doctors must be trained every year to beat the crisis.'[xix]

The following month, Sir Alan Langlands announced that the NHS needed to achieve an increase in productivity unparalleled in its fifty-year history, in order to keep up with hospital waiting lists. One wonders if he is familiar with the old adage about flogging a dead horse.

How important is it that doctors are subjected to ever-increasing mountains of paperwork? Well, in a report covered by *USA Today* it was found that Boomers (i.e. the age group containing many of the doctors currently in practice) would actually *pay money* in order to simplify their lives.[xx] The statistics ran as follows after the question was posed as to whether they would accept a smaller pay cheque in exchange for having a simpler lifestyle:

age group	agree
18 – 34	33%
35 – 49	41%
50 – 64	34%
65 plus	15%

Don't Waste Doctors

The DWD (Don't Waste Doctors) Investigation of May 1998 was a three-year study carried out in Manchester by two doctors and a research assistant. It was started because 32 per cent of hospital senior house officer jobs remained unfilled in the North West of England. Of the 3,805 medical graduates studied, it was found that 24 per cent were no longer working for the NHS two years after qualifying and of these, 40 per cent said they did not wish to return. Among reasons given were:

- Poor working conditions
- Appalling physical environment
- Poor morale among staff
- Long hours, poor representation and unfair responsibilities

It currently costs around £200,000 to train a doctor and this high rate of wastage also represents a loss of many years of training and dissipation of skills available to the country. The BMA reckons that in 1998, 8 per cent of newly qualified doctors left during their first year!

There is no doubt whatsoever that this disillusionment and lack of morale is a direct result of poor leadership. In order to be able to administer anything efficiently, one needs to be a good leader, and in order to lead, one needs respect and credibility. This is not always present, as the following will demonstrate.

Are They Trying To Tell Her Something?

The following is something experienced by one of the authors, who, prior to this episode, had not considered that the job of being his secretary was regarded as a 'punishment posting'. Perhaps it isn't – the reader must decide as to whether the rest of this woman's experience constitutes even fair and reasonable treatment – it certainly does not fall under the heading of inspired leadership!

She began her working life as a medical secretary, and worked her way up the grades, acquiring skills and experience. She then sought promotion, and obtained a post in medical personnel. Sadly, this is often the only way for a medical secretary to gain further promotion and pay – by moving into another field. It does not necessarily make her a bad person! And then she became pregnant. In those days, it wasn't as easy (perhaps it still isn't) to return to her post and she reverted to being a medical secretary. And there she stayed, quite happily performing her task in an efficient manner. She then fell foul of her former administrative colleagues. After various forays into the 'let us make this job difficult so she will leave' game, she was presented with this work plan.

First, she was to be the medical secretary to one of the authors, and if she turned down this job, she would be out.

Second, she would have to move hospitals.

She had worked for many years at one of the town's two hospitals – it was convenient as she lived within walking distance, could return home at lunchtime to tend her elderly mother and collect her children from school. Unfortunately, the author works at the town's other hospital, several miles away. So, the plan was that she should get on the hospital shuttle each morning (for she had to accept this post) and get to his hospital for 9.30 am, work there for three hours and then get the return shuttle. Thus she puts in five days of three hours' duration. But she is paid for thirty. How is this squared? Why, she is expected to walk back to her previous hospital after lunch and sit in reception (not working at the reception desk or doing anything useful), yes, sit in reception twiddling her thumbs until her leaving time.

It will not be lost on the reader that the author has, since her appointment, been denied secretarial services for a great number of hours per week. Fortunately, and this may come as a surprise to our readers, his letters are very short!

Hospital managers are clearly poor leaders. They have tried to command respect by demonstrations of political power, and thought that by suspending consultants, they would intimidate those remaining. Doctors have not been frightened by this, but have become more entrenched. But it has lowered morale. The greatest commodity of the old NHS was the dedication and the enthusiasm of its workers. Before the Revolution, hospitals used to be happy and good places to work.

Inept, heavy-handed leadership skills based on a market economy have killed the goose that laid the golden egg, and it can probably never be resurrected. Removal of resources and concomitant bullying by managers of nurses, porters and others who actually *work* in hospitals, together with a total lack of communication (oral or otherwise) has meant that the morale which was once its greatest asset has continued to decline so that we are in a situation where there may be an overabundance of Stasi but doctors are leaving in droves, and those who remain cannot wait to retire at an early age.

Failings in leadership are not confined to hospital managers (though they may be thought to have a virtual monopoly!). A case was reported in *Hospital Doctor* of a junior doctor who, through the stress of overwork took to drugs, which he obtained by falsifying entries in the controlled drug register where he worked. The judge concluded, 'You were plainly suffering from stress and we understand that.' He was sentenced to 100 hours' community service.[xxi]

Of course, we would all like to feel that we ourselves ran happy departments and were supportive of our colleagues, etc. But we must of course be cautious when interpreting reports of how people do actually manage their departments. At a commemorative lecture we attended, the late great doctor and his legacy were praised. Amongst the glowing testimonies from former juniors was the remark: 'Everyone was considered equal. Monthly, he would convene a meeting at which everyone had to be present.'

No doubt it was easier for some than others to manage to be there.

CHAPTER 3

LIONS DRIVEN BY DONKEYS[1]

Should the Blind Lead the Myopic?

Richard J Daley, mayor of Chicago from 1955 until 1976 was known as the 'last of the big-city bosses'. It was he who said: 'The police of the City of Chicago are not there to create order, but to preserve the existing disorder.'

It is a strange phenomenon but well known to any who (like the authors) spend time reading medical journals of the past, that

---

[1] The title of this chapter was the original title of this book: it is taken from a conversation reported in the Great War Memoirs of General Erich von Falkenhayn, (1861–1922) Chief of the Imperial German Staff. Erich Friedrich Wilhelm Ludendorff, (1865–1937) Prussian General who was mainly responsible for Germany's military policy and strategy in the latter years of World War I commented during a hard fought battle that, 'The English soldiers fight like lions!'

His Chief of Staff, General Max Hoffmann (1869–1927), widely regarded as one of the finest German staff officers and greatest tacticians of the imperial period, sagely replied, 'True. But don't we know that they are lions led by donkeys?'

On reflection we opted to change this, and the word 'led' was replaced because of course at present there is absolutely no leadership within the NHS. Alan Clark wrote a book in 1961 called *The Donkeys*, about the British Army Officers in the Great War.

there are few things in medicine (and medical politics) which are entirely new. Take for example the Address of the President of the American Surgical Association for 1908, William H Carmalt:

> Hospital directors or trustees find it difficult to appreciate this feature of hospital management; most of them regard anything that does not directly (according to their light) concern the immediate welfare of the individual patient as unnecessary expense, a waste of trust funds.[i]

Once more it would seem that the Americans have beaten us to it. Perhaps, however, this can be updated by adding, 'does not directly alter the waiting lists or any other factor which might influence their bonuses.' There is, of course, a neat inversion in the logic that it is the administrative staff that needs to be provided, as part of their remunerative package[2], with cars and expensive offices, pot plants, etc. No doubt some management guru has ordained that more and higher quality work is produced as a result of conducive surroundings. On the other hand, Thorstein Veblen[3] has said that nobody travelling on a business trip would ever have been missed if he did not arrive. One obviously has to carefully select whom one is going to quote if the decor of one's workplace needs improvement. High quality management needs to be recruited, and, it seems, the only way to do this is by offering high salaries[4]. What of the doctors and nurses? This argument has been heard before in

---

[2]That is to say, pay.

[3]Your authors have *not* made this name up.

[4]'Gold is the key, whatever else we try.' Molière's *School for Wives*, 1662.

political circles: if wages are too high, then the will to work is taken away and absenteeism increases – they can get by with working less – i.e. there is no drive to work overtime, etc. Yet the same people come out with the idea of high rewards being necessary to recompense hard work and attract the right calibre of recruit. If one looks for consistency in life, especially in political life, one is likely to be disappointed. Your authors can be consistent on this point. In summary, to ask the administration whether the offices etc, are necessary is like asking a barber about the advisability of a haircut. The lay public often has a good insight into the relative value of having people specifically to perform administrative duties:

> Once upon a time the administrators had upset him but ever since the day we worked out mathematically the functions of the various people in an organization and those of the administrators came out consistently zero he had been gleefully immune.[ii]

There are, of course, certain aspects of life, death, and disease which, for better or worse, are experienced at first hand only by doctors and nurses. The Stasi can only at second hand have much insight into this, and that may well explain a lot in itself. There has always been the gifted writer who can convey some of the awfulness of serious or chronic disease, and, for those who wish, this can be a means by which the demands of those in the caring professions and the constraints of the bean-counters can be understood.

Leonard Kriegel, who ended up as Professor of English at the City College of the City University in New York (one might say that he was a person who relished a challenge!) writes in an entirely non self-pitying way of his contraction of polio during the epidemic which swept the eastern United States during the summer of 1944. He was at that time eleven years old, and had to spend two years in the appropriately named New York State Reconstruction Home in West Haverstraw. Following initial diagnosis, patients were kept in isolation for a period of ten days to two weeks, and then subjected to as much heat as they could stand – both with 'hot packs' and immersion in hot water. Any recovery of muscle use usually took place within these three months.... After ten months, he stood for the first time, with the aid of callipers; he then spent an hour daily for the next six months in the rehabilitation room, learning how to climb steps and manipulate his crutches.[iii] Six months! Why, with a little (free) enterprise that could be reduced to a day-case procedure with callipers sponsored by Dynorod!

The counter argument might be that only someone distanced from the 'coal-face' of death and disease is likely to have the necessary objectivity for making important decisions. Too detailed knowledge may impinge on the ability to weigh up all conflicting claims. On the other hand, ignorance has often led to the most bizarre decisions being made. For example, during the Second World War, a politician who had been given the task of harbouring the nation's resources as Minister of Food learnt that the energy value of water was nothing. Her considered opinion was that all bread should therefore be converted to toast which, weight for weight, would contain more energy! George Eliot, in *Middlemarch* describes the problem nicely:

A liberal education had of course left him free to read the indecent passages in the school classics, but beyond a general sense of secrecy and obscenity in connection with his internal structure, had left his imagination quite unbiased, so that for anything he knew his brains lay in small bags at his temples and he had no more thought of representing to himself how his blood circulated than how paper served instead of gold.

Muddling Through

In early 1939, Lord Horder said: 'We are a pragmatic race. We make things work even when they seem, by theory, to be unworkable. We shall probably do the same with our health services.'[iv]

Aneurin Bevan's widow, Jenny Lee MP, also implied that the pre-NHS health service was always in a bit of a muddle: 'Many of us have associations with the between-the-wars health service; a great patchwork, a good deal of good intentions, a great deal of inadequacies.'[v]

The main muddler in the hospital before the NHS was the Medical Superintendent, but after his overthrow and demise by the drain sniffers (see Cogwheel), the job of fudging went to the hospital secretary (he was the shabbily-dressed fellow who always had a cigarette burning). Before the Revolution, he muddled on very adequately and heroically (with, believe it or not, the support of the consultants). The first major restructuring of 1974 is usually attributed to Barbara Castle (see also Red Cow, Chapter 2), but in fact it had been mainly orchestrated by Sir Keith Joseph, her Tory predecessor, and as our readers might imagine was not very exciting. There was another 'damp squib'[vi] called the Merrison Report in 1979[5] and in 1982 another Tory attempt at re-arranging the deckchairs on the Titanic with the

---

[5]Sir Alex Merrison, Vice-Chancellor of the University of Bristol himself admitted his report had 'no blinding revelation which would transform the NHS'.

highly innovative and original title *Patients First*[6]. Not a lot happened, however, until 1983 and the Griffiths Report.[vii]

You may remember that Brian Salmon, the author of the Salmon report (which was the death knell for nurses) was the managing director of J Lyons (the tea-room people). Well, Roy Griffiths had quite a lot in common. He too was, of course, not medically qualified but was the deputy managing director of Sainsbury the supermarket chain. Norman Fowler was the Minister of Health and the whole ethos of Mrs Thatcher's administration was that of the marketplace. Like most members of the Iron Lady's cabinet, Norman Fowler liked to keep her happy, and probably thought that she would be very happy indeed if he asked a grocer how to run the NHS (she was the daughter of a Grantham greengrocer). Evidently Roy Griffiths spent quite a lot of time during the preparation of his report dining with the consultants from St Thomas' Hospital. It is the opinion of the authors that this does not *necessarily* make him into a bad person, particularly as he himself had no medical background and therefore could not realistically be expected to know the implications of St Thomas[7].

It was Griffiths' lack of ever having worked in a hospital which not only made him so eminently suitable for the job, but also made him so blissfully unaware of the highly informal 'cocktail party' lines of communication and power which had always existed in that service. Griffiths just could not comprehend or accept what appeared to him to be a complete absence of any management structure (which of course had always been a

---

[6]Consultative Paper on Structure and Management of NHS. HMSO, 1979.

[7]On a sideline (unusual for us!), St Thomas' in Oxford was a penitentiary 'where women of frail morals are kept under surveillance'!

prerequisite for the running of grocery shops). It was Roy Griffiths who gave us the famous line:

> If Florence Nightingale was carrying her lamp through the corridors of the NHS today, she would almost certainly be searching for the people in charge.

He therefore suggested lots and lots of administrators, preferably with experience of retailing. Mrs Thatcher loved his proposals. She concurred with him that the difference between the care of the nation's health and the economic management of a chain store is inconsequential; clearly the principles are the same. Neither did either of them concede or even realise that general management by untrained personnel is inappropriate for the hospital service where the main 'commodity for sale' is the knowledge, experience and technical skills of professional (and often pompous and self-opinionated) consultants and nurses who might not take kindly to school leavers telling them how to organise their operating theatres.

Griffiths also upset the drain sniffers, who since Cogwheel had seen themselves in the lead role. That, after all, is why they had ousted the Medical Superintendents. Griffiths upset the nurses, who had been fighting a valiant rear-guard action since Salmon had almost totally disempowered them; now they were totally crushed. Florence Nightingale had succeeded in securing a power base for nurses by nurses, but this was now completely overturned by Griffiths' new odious and despicable concept of a Chief Executive Officer who would be non-medical, non-nursing and a complete autocrat within the hospital.

Although there are differences of opinion as to the timing of the Revolution, there is little doubt that the implementation of the Griffiths Report certainly marked its consolidation. In fact, in a book by Webster[8] in 1998 on the political history of the NHS, he likens the perpetual revolution Mrs Thatcher introduced as a result of the Griffiths Report to that of Chairman Mao.[viii]

As time went by it became apparent that 'more output' was being demanded with more and more operations needed, and ever higher bed occupancy figures. It came to the point that some doctors were sufficiently concerned with the quality of their own service to stop promising to see or operate on more patients than they knew they could deal with. This was essential to avoid mounting delay in consultation and treatment for all of them – 'he gives twice as much good who gives quickly'[9]. This was a rejection of the peculiarly British form of fraudulent promise known as the 'waiting list.'[10] It gave the responsibility for the volume of service to the purse holders and manpower controllers. The 'management' found this tacit acknowledgement

---

[8]Charles Webster, the Director of the Wellcome History of Medicine Unit and Senior Research Fellow at All Soul's College, Oxford was once a school master at Sheffield City Grammar School, where he was the form master of one of the authors.

[9]*Inopi beneficium bis dat, qui dat celeriter.* Attributed to Seneca.

[10]As any costermonger knows, if supply matches demand there can be no 'waiting list'; there may, but should not, be a backlog like that which maintains the cachet of Morgan cars. If demand exceeds supply, and is concealed in a waiting list, then a runaway disparity exists that only reaches equilibrium when the reduction by death or despair equals the increase by the excess of promise over performance. This results in delay for all and a curious equality in which no one is satisfied. Clinical priority may or may not be lost. In the 1950s, as their non-emergency operating lists escalated, surgeons were obliged to stream them, in categories like: A – needs doing most, can and will be done first. B – Should be done if space after A, and just might with some windfall facility for which I am lobbying. C – Desirable in a different world but cannot and will not be done in my foreseeable circumstances. C, of course, grew the longest, and would therefore have become the target of the, happily then not yet invented, 'waiting list initiative'.

that any part of the shop was 'Sold Out' much more offensive than they did consultants who acquiesced in the waiting list fraud for the purposes of stimulating private practice – for, as we were to discover later, the management motto was 'Patients First'. The Stasi aggregated waiting lists as the anonymous responsibility of newly recruited layers of management, who bought lots of expensive computers to put them on. They then indulged in highly publicised, costly, ineffective and ill-directed short term patches known as 'waiting list initiatives', motivated by political number massaging and ignoring clinical priority. Intrinsic delay continued, the clinician in the front line continued to bear the brunt of complaints, and the patients, as always, to suffer with astonishingly little complaint.

What is perhaps amazing is that medical opposition was by no means unanimous, and in 1988 some doctors apparently welcomed the changes. Dr Peter Bruggen, author of *Who Cares* wrote:

I welcomed the bold heralding of this revolution because I thought the whole thing needed a very good shake up. I thought doctors did have too much power and did not use it well. The profession had learned to manage all sorts of elaborate interventions and treatments, but not outpatient clinics or waiting lists.[ix]

Enthoven's Contribution

Shortly after Griffiths had been asked to make intelligent suggestions about the restructuring of the NHS, along the lines of buying and selling large quantities of doughnuts and employing surgeons and theatre sisters in a similar manner perhaps to employing school leavers to stack baked beans or fill old ladies shopping baskets, the Private Hospital sector did not wish to appear to lag behind. The Nuffield Provincial Hospitals Trust, presumably unable to find anyone from the local supermarket or fast-food restaurant to help them out, did the next best thing and invited President Johnson's former Assistant Secretary of State for Defense to give his views on the NHS. His name was Alain C Enthoven and in 1985 he published *Reflections on the Management of the NHS*.[x] Whereas Roy Griffiths had done his homework by dining with consultants from the large teaching hospital in Lambeth, Enthoven chose to dine with politicians. Actually he *lunched* with two of Mrs Thatcher's acolytes: John Redwood and David Willetts. It is therefore surprising that his report proved so insightful.

He thought that the NHS was caught in an almost inextricable gridlock of forces. He also said: 'Politicians can use performance indicators for "number games" that destroy credibility.'

He said that an HMO (Health Maintenance Organisation) should have leading it 'a doctor whose leadership is accepted by other doctors to organize and control the delivery of services.' He added one or two more thoughts about medical leadership, pointing out that leaders have to enjoy the respect of those led. He advocated the need for 'a prestigious consultant with knowledge and instincts for management' to lead the HMOs but acknowledged that nobody would be likely to take the job on. Evidently the Iron Lady liked the Enthoven Report, but why, you might well ask, did nothing ever come of it? Well in fact quite a few of the other recommendations in it formed the basis of Mrs Thatcher's 1991 reforms. She left out Enthoven's excellent suggestions about the most appropriate leaders and Lee-Potter says that:

By cherry-picking what appealed to her market instincts and

ignoring questions of coherence, scale and suitability to Britain's healthcare (sic) system, and by allowing Kenneth Clarke to dismiss Enthoven's strong recommendation for the limited trial of ideas, she jeopardized much of the huge progress that the health service has made since 1948.

Enthoven paid a second visit to the UK in 1989, and he pointed out on that occasion that a successful relationship between administrator and the professionals remains the single most important unresolved factor in the NHS. As he put it, if doctors do not trust management, 'Then forget it.'[xi] The old Scottish proverb immediately springs to mind: 'Trust not a new friend, nor an old enemy.'[xii]

Confrontation

Thus as a result of Griffiths, the Stasi moved in. Consensus was replaced by confrontation. The idealism of the doctors was replaced by stifling management practices from Sainsbury's. Professional commitment of the health service workers[11] (not only doctors and nurses but also physiotherapists, radiographers, laboratory technicians, audiologists, porters, telephonists and kitchen staff) was driven into the ground as outdated. The nine-to-five culture was to replace dedication and staying behind after work for the good of the patients and for the benefit of the service. Efficiency was to replace effectiveness. Goodwill and morale were made obsolete and élitist. The NHS was now to be a commercial concern and not a charity.

What is particularly sad is that Enthoven had repeatedly specifically suggested that small pilot studies should be

---

[11]In this context your authors do not include administrators as *workers*.

undertaken, but Mrs Thatcher and her hatchet-man (Kenneth Clarke) were not in favour of this. The BMA suggested that the new market economy schemes of the purchaser-provider split, Fund Holding General Practices and NHS Trust Hospitals be tried in one or two regions first. For some reason East Anglia was suggested, though we do not know what the inhabitants had done wrong to receive this treatment. Kenneth Clarke would have none of this pussyfooting and wanted to bulldoze his reforms through. He looked upon the BMA as 'those lefties from Tavistock Square'[12], and told them 'you buggers will sabotage it!' The BMA did in fact try to do this, and embarked on an expensive plan to undermine the new proposals including advertising posters showing a steamroller and the caption 'Mrs Thatcher's proposals for the NHS. Don't let her steamroller the White Paper through.' Other posters and adverts were even more vituperative – the very first said: 'Mr Clarke wants to introduce a new spirit of cooperation in the NHS – the health of the patient vs. the cost of the treatment'. Another read: 'The NHS – under funded, undermined, under threat'. The last in the series was: 'What do you call a man who ignores medical advice? – Mr Clarke'.

Mistrust of management grew[13]. It was certainly not helped when a document from the Trent Regional Health Authority (amongst the most draconian) was leaked: it invited the Stasi of

---

[12]BMA House, the HQ of the British Medical Association, is in Tavistock Square, London WC14.

[13]'The Camel Who Shat In The River' was one of Aesop's original 'coarse and brutal' fables (not the popular ones prized by the Victorians; it can be found in Robert & Olivia Temple's *Aesop's Fables*, Penguin Classics: 'A camel was crossing a swiftly-flowing stream. He shat and immediately saw his own dung floating in front of him, carried by the rapidity of the current. "What is that there?" he asked himself. "That which was behind me I now see pass in front of me." Moral: 'This applies to a situation where the rabble and the idiots hold sway rather than the eminent and the sensible.'

the new Trust Hospitals to discipline dissidents, whom it called 'renegades, subversives and opposers' and it actually said:

> If a self-governing trust values teamwork, it needs to confront the obstructive and the prima donna and when all else has failed to persuade individuals to sign up to a corporate philosophy.[xiii]

Prima donnas might have come to epitomise getting up the nose of one's co-workers but no opera company has (to your authors' knowledge) been as hell-bent on self-destruction as to recommend their extermination. As Dr Lee-Potter pointed out: 'The so-called "corporate philosophy" for medicine was voiced a long time ago – by Hippocrates!'[xiv]

A Damn Bad Business[14]

So, in 1991, the Chief Executive Officers started to be appointed to the NHS Trusts in large numbers. The applicants saw the opportunities provided by the exorbitantly high salaries. The most unlikely people were set on. Overnight it seemed that the man who used to sharpen the used hypodermic needles in the hospital basement was now a Chief Executive! The Trusts could not always find failures from supermarkets or tea-rooms and so appointed all other manner of second-rate businessmen. Bus firm managers, haulage contractors and laundry managers were welcomed with open arms. There were very few doctors.

Whilst knowing of hardly any doctors being appointed to such

---

[14]The name of a very readable book (1997) by Jeremy Lee-Potter, haematologist husband of *Daily Mail* columnist Lynda. He borrowed the title from a quote by Sir Humphrey Rolleston: 'Medicine is a noble profession, but a damn bad business.'

exalted positions, we can relate the fascinating saga of an old army chum of theirs. Colonel Richard qualified in medicine and joined the Army as a regimental medical officer. He went on to train as an ENT surgeon, but since he had an eye for the main chance and saw that the best opportunities for promotion lay in administration, he left surgery and took that up. The good colonel had obtained post-graduate degrees in public health and also in management. He had gone on to become Commanding Officer of a large military hospital in Germany. He had also done medical administrative jobs in the United Kingdom, but had retired from HM Forces at the relatively early age of fifty-three. Understandably, he thought he would apply for one of the new CEO posts. He had made the presumption that because he was not only a doctor, but also had additional qualifications in public health and management, he would be eminently suitable and stand a good chance.

He was not even short-listed!

The job went to an accountant who had no further qualifications. Clearly a doctor as CEO would be a terrible threat to the new system of internal marketing. Because he was a member of a caring profession, he might let his Hippocratic training influence market considerations. The fact that he had successfully commanded a hospital in the past was presumably another disadvantage. It was clear to a blind Trust Chairman on a galloping horse that he was certainly not suitable for the job.

Let us see then what type of people the new CEOs were. It has been shown that they were not from the caring professions of medicine and nursing; they were not even the orthodox types of civil servant.

Stark Naked Civil Servants
Whether they like to admit it or not, the Stasi are civil servants

74

(and for that matter, so are consultants, GPs and nurses[15]). Most civil servants have to take a series of graded examinations: the Inland Revenue, for example, has a very hierarchical rank structure and passing a written examination is a necessary prerequisite before ascending the ladder of promotion. Even the Post Office has a series of exams and before a bog standard postman can be promoted to a post person (higher grade) (PHG) he too has to take a written examination. These examinations concentrate mainly on subjects relevant respectively to taxation and postal communications. The Stasi, however, do not have any similar hoops to jump through, and can easily command very highly paid jobs without ever taking a written examination. In addition to their specialist subjects, other civil servants also have instruction and take examinations in what is known in the Army as 'staff work'. Indeed in all parts of the civil service, this sort of work is the very bread and butter of administration.

Efficient management relies almost entirely on communication and staff work lays down the guidelines for communication within the civil service. It includes the correct way to write the different types of letters (formal letters, demi-official or DO and routine letters), when to write a letter and when to send a memo (whether or not to sign a memo), how to write a service paper, how to write the agenda or the minutes of a meeting, etc. In this regard, we are amazed at the staff work at regional and national level and consider the standard as 'woeful'. The total lack of any structural vocational training is perhaps best underlined by the appointment in the North of England of one chief executive who had never actually worked in a hospital before, but was the manager of a bus company!

---

[15]Arranged in alphabetical order rather than for any other reason.

A new Chief Executive Officer was appointed to a District General Hospital in 1998 at an enormous starting salary. It is worthy of note that when a consultant from a neighbouring hospital was told of the appointment, he did not ask 'Which hospital is she from?', but 'Has she worked in hospitals before, or is she from outside?'

The proper use of English is encouraged by most branches of the Civil Service, but it almost appears to be actively discouraged by the upper echelons of the Stasi. One of us once found five mistakes in a seven-line memo. They tend to send memos all the time, usually inappropriately, but it appears that no one has ever told them when to send a memo or when a letter. Sending a memorandum also sidesteps the thorny problem of using a salutation. A CEO, for example, would avoid the highly contentious 'Dear Colleague' trap, and those with a chip on their shoulder[16] would never have to address a consultant as 'Sir'.

With respect to *procedure* they appear to be similarly clueless. Our readers will doubtless have perceived that the authors of this book are diplomatic and tolerant men who would not go out of their way to 'rattle the cage' of their friendly local Stasi (perish the thought!). Sadly, one of your authors had presumably upset no less a personage than the Director of Internal Audit[17]. As he remembers he had caused offence to this woman by asking her if she were medically qualified. Seriously offended, she informed him that as a result of this derisive and provocative remark (his exact words were 'Are you medically

---

[16]The question has arisen in the minds of your authors: 'Is a well-balanced hospital administrator one with a chip on both shoulders?'

[17]The Stasispeak for highly paid NHS accountant.

qualified?') she would report his insolent and scurrilous behaviour and 'institute a Complaints Procedure against him'. Totally intimidated, he almost forbore to point out that only a patient or the relative of a patient could properly take out a complaints procedure against him (or even *institute* one as she had said). He thought, however, he had better mention this fact and then told her, with all the diplomacy, tact and forbearing he could muster, that he thought she would be better employed venting her spleen on him by *instituting* a Grievance Procedure (which is the NHS practice for one employee to officially complain about the conduct of another). For some reason, at this point, she put the phone down on him.

Nonetheless the Director of Personnel (whose nickname in the hospital was 'A-level', because he didn't have one) made an appointment to see the author a week later, and although a generous-minded reader might have reasonably assumed that the Director of Personnel of a District General Hospital might well be expected to know the difference, he too made the self same error. 'I'm afraid Ms X has instituted [yes, he said it too!] a Complaints Procedure against you.' The whole thing fell into abeyance (presumably because asking anyone if they are a doctor cannot be considered to be really grievous).

Chinese Whispers

Another example of the ludicrous practices of the Stasi concerns what is done when a patient makes an official complaint. When we outlined this procedure to a pal who is a lawyer, he laughed until tears ran down his cheeks! Quite honestly, he could not believe that it actually takes place. It is left to our readers, who it is assumed must be of a discerning character to have acquired this book and read thus far, to make up their own minds, but they are assured of its veracity and the fact it is actually practised with gravitas throughout the NHS.

Any complaint to the Chief Executive is given to the Complaints Facilitator who then writes to all the nursing staff and medical staff for their comments. If the doctors and nurses are silly enough to respond, the Facilitator writes a draft letter and presents it to the CEO for signature. A letter is then sent to the complainant signed by a person who has most probably never spoken to any of the players in the tragedy. The writer of the letter (but not the signatory) has spent many man-hours questioning doctors and nurses (who for the most part accede) and then puts together a second-hand version of the facts. The Chinese Whispers scenario then continues if the Chief Executive decides to alter it.

When the poor complainant receives his letter from the Chief Executive, certain false conclusions are understandably made. First, Joe Public will assume from the subscription of the signatory that it is from a very important and responsible member of the hospital staff. Secondly, he may well believe that the information contained in the letter is accurate. It is most unlikely that he will know that it is not only hearsay, but second-hand hearsay (hearsay of hearsay!).

Leading on from the incompetence of correct procedure, we would like to give an example of actual managerial stupidity by the Stasi. In June 1998, in a hospital in the West Midlands, an edict went out to all consultants telling them that in future they must not under any circumstances cancel any outpatient clinics without four weeks' notice. The consultants receiving this high-handed missive were then told that it was mandatory that they attend a meeting to discuss this matter at a date one week from the receipt of the letter – not five weeks from receipt, but one!

What a masterpiece of mismanagement! This is not an isolated example: many, many more could be cited but your authors do not wish to appear to be whingeing. They would certainly not want it to be thought that this chapter had been written to discredit the Stasi, and would also not wish to engender any reference whatsoever to a 'booze-up at a brewery'!

Showdown at the Little Chef

So much for the specialized training and high level performance of the Stasi, but what sort of people are they at heart? This story may seem incredible, but was told by a retired general who had become Chairman of a Healthcare Trust[18]. He confided that he was quite abashed by it and seriously wondered about what sort of organization he had joined. It all took place when the first wave of Healthcare Trusts was in full sway and this poor Chief Executive had been unable to convince the consultants at his hospital, or the GPs, or the Community Health Council, or the District Council (or anybody else for that matter) that this was a good idea.

His regional bosses decided that he would have to move on! It is not the fact that his bosses sacked him, but the manner in which they did it that is worthy of mention. It is also ironic that only a short time before his dismissal, this particular toad of an administrator had appeared on regional television saying that he was going to sack one of the surgical consultants at his hospital if he didn't start to toe the line[19].

---

[18] It is interesting that he did not stay in this post for long and left it after only eighteen months or so to do similar sort of work in the United States – he became the director of an armaments firm.

[19] That consultant is still in post, despite a temporary suspension twenty years later!

He himself came from Glasgow and his regional boss was a compatriot; she was a powerful Scottish woman who insisted on the title *Ms*[20] and did not take kindly to people who pronounced it 'manuscript' (for a note on Scots GSoH see footnote 15 in the Whistleblowers entry in chapter 2). She was Chairman of the Regional Health Authority, but demanded that her underlings referred to her as a chair![21] One of your authors is a life member of the Queen's English Society and therefore could never really in all conscience refer to anyone as a chair. But once again we digress. The Scots 'Chair' had clearly decided that

If it were done when 'tis done, then t'were well
It were done quickly[xv]

and so she rang him up. She evidently had some minor degree of decorum because she didn't sack him by telephone: she asked him to drive to a roadside café some forty miles away from his

---

[20]Your authors are at a loss to help the reader in this matter (i.e. the suggested pronunciation of Ms). Obviously only those rare persons with iron self-control can possibly say 'muzz' without at worst laughing out loud, or at best giggling. 'Manuscript' is perhaps somewhat provocative; the best suggestion is that 'Miss' said quickly is always courteous and polite, and has the great advantage that one does not feel silly.

[21]Those readers who have had the boon of a classical education will remember no doubt declining the first declension feminine noun *mensa* (which for the benefit of any administrators who are *still* reading this book means 'table' and has nothing at all to do with the egg-head boffin society with high IQs who get endless hours of pleasure from tricky puzzles with geometric shapes). Those ancient Romans were obviously terribly clever, as anyone who has declined *mensa* will know, because *mensa* not only represents the nominative case, but also the vocative, and was extremely useful if one ever wished to talk to, or address a table; you may remember it meant '*O table*'. Incidentally, Winston Churchill's first thrashing at Harrow was evidently because he called into question the wisdom of learning the Latin for how to address a table.

DGH. He drove himself there and she was driven there (again some forty miles) by her chauffeur. Then in the Little Chef over a cosy cup of tea on a Formica table she tactfully broke the news that he should clear his desk.[22] Such evidently is the professionalism of the higher echelons of the regional administration! She was then whisked back to Regional HQ by her driver, whilst the crestfallen Chief Executive drove home.

Prima Non Nocere

So far we have examined the extensive special vocational training programmes of the Stasi which no doubt leads to the amazing competence in management skills achieved by the 'fat controllers'[23] of the NHS. An important question, however, which begs an answer is, 'What exactly do modern-day Stasi actually do?' In the past, the harassed-looking man with the Woodbine[24] supervised cooks, cleaners and wage clerks; nowadays these very essential jobs are considered *infra dig*[25] for modern Stasi and delegated to minions. Therefore the question remains – what useful purpose do they now serve?

Sadly, we have been unable to find any answer to this poser.

---

[22]To hit someone in the nose without any prior warning is known in Yorkshire as a 'Scarborough Warning'. This form of surprise attack evidently takes its name from the naval bombardment of Scarborough by the German fleet in early August 1914, when the bewildered inhabitants of that fair town had barely realised that war had been declared!

[23]Apologies here to the wonderful stories by the Rev W Awdry.

[24]Wild Woodbines were estimable but cheap unfiltered cigarettes made by W D and H O Wills. They came in a green packet with an excellent design and were smoked illicitly by your authors, not behind the chicken sheds, but in the school lavs!

[25]For any administrator *still* persevering, *infra* means below in Latin, and *dig* is a shortened form of dignitatem or dignity; hence below one's dignity, or derogatory.

One might try to solve the enigma by examining whether or not there would be any significant change if the Stasi were removed. The answer is a resounding and very definite 'yes'.

If they were all sacked, matters would certainly improve.

This can be seen to some extent at the weekend, when no Stasi are to be seen anywhere in the hospital buildings, and things definitely seem to run smoother. The lost morale would undoubtedly return quite quickly if all the Stasi were taken out. It could therefore be concluded that they have a negative sort of role. Your authors will at this point once again digress slightly, but only for the point of illustration; dear reader, do not think we have taken leave of our senses when we begin to talk of Karl Marx. He held that the difference between a pile of pieces of wood and a newly completed chair[26] was the work and skill of the carpenter, whose contribution was the 'added value'. We like to think of the current set up in hospitals as being like a car factory: labour is added to steel, glass, rubber, etc (all of which have a cost) – and the result is a Lada worth less than this cost. The Stasi have managed to take money, resources, labour and goodwill – and end up with a service less than the total of its components.

There is a fundamental medical principle (attributed to Hippocrates) of *Prima non nocere*, or 'Above all, do not inflict harm'. In essence, Hippocrates was implying that if you cannot do any positive good for you patient, it is better to do nothing than to interfere in a meddlesome manner and end up by making matters worse. A simple example of this would be the use of a steroid skin ointment for a case of scabies, athlete's foot or nappy rash. The steroid would not only not help, it would make things worse.

---

[26]History books are vague as to whether he actually ever uttered the words 'O chair', in Latin or any other language.

The Stasi have never cottoned onto the *prima non nocere* idea. They just cannot let things lie – even when they are working well. Probably the underlying cause for this officious meddlesomeness is their unjustifiably exorbitant salary (See Chapter 5, Fees and Remuneration). An orthopaedic surgeon was once overheard in a medical executive meeting (during the boring meaningless drone of a Chief Executive) asking his colleague 'Why don't they pay her to stay at home?' But if your basic pay is a good deal more than that of a consultant orthopaedic surgeon, you may feel that you *ought* to somehow try (however ineptly) to justify the taxpayers' outlay. You come to work to meddle, albeit with the best will in the world.

A series of booklets on management called 'The One Minute Manager' swept America in the 1980s, suggesting that the most effective managers only work two hours a week, leaving the people alone most of the time to work effectively themselves. A sage old headmaster at the Sheffield City Grammar School often quoted the words 'Satan finds' to one of your authors. At the time, that author was somewhat perplexed as to what was meant. He has since discovered that it is from Isaac Watt's poem 'Agaynste Idlenesse'. The full quote is:

For Satan finds some mischiefe stille,
For idle handes to doe.

Thus the Stasi make changes for the sake of something to do, to fill in all the unnecessary time they spend at work, to justify their non-jobs. Instead, it would be better for everyone if they stayed at home and never came to the hospital – or only ever held meetings (which would amount to the same thing).

The changes they make are often ludicrous. This gives rise to a cyclical form of activity. Another Paul Pry[27] will in due course come along, and return things to what they were originally – taking credit for this 'innovation'!

We have heard colleagues suggest that nobody would notice if these grey non-entities did not come to work – nobody would miss them. This premise is strongly contested; we are definitely of the opinion that if the Stasi did not come to work, everyone would certainly notice, because things would start to get better!

To Kill an Admiral[28]

A few months after the Glaswegian received his mittimus[29], he was replaced by a bright young lady accountant.

It was in the South-West where our friend and colleague, Surgeon Vice-Admiral Sir Godfrey Milton Thompson exposed to what outrageous levels this Petticoat Power had penetrated[30]. Sir Godfrey retired from the Royal Navy in 1991 after thirty-five years as a medical officer. He was appointed to the post of Chairman of the Cornwall Community Healthcare Trust, and furthermore was a highly successful appointment (which might be said to be unusual

---

[27]Paul Pry – the archetypal stereotype for an idle, meddlesome fellow came from a character in a play by John Poole in which Paul Pry had no occupation of his own and consequently always interfered with other folks' business.

[28]The quotation is much more famous for its ending: '*Dans ce pays-ci il est bon de tuer de temps en temps un amiral pour encourager les autres?*' which for the sake of our non-francophone readers translates as follows: 'In this country [England] it is thought well to kill an admiral from time to time to encourage the others?'

[29]A posh colloquial way of saying 'got the sack'. Interestingly, shortly afterwards, he was appointed to another Chief Executive post at the other end of England!

[30]We initially wrote 'pernicious Petticoat Power' but thought it might be overdoing alliteration's artful aid a little too much.

in itself on two counts: first, chairmen are not usually competent at all, and second, because they are not usually doctors[31]). In the early nineties, the Health Secretary was Virginia Bottomley, and the NHS had unashamedly stated its overtly sexist policy of positive discrimination in favour of women. Clearly it had been considered that it was quite acceptable in this particular case (in the same was that it is obviously not wrong to have a racist TV programme called 'Black Matters' but it would be provocative and unacceptable to have a show called 'Caucasian Matters'[32]). Also around this time, the Cornwall Community Healthcare Trust was going to merge with a hospital to form a bigger new Trust with a slightly altered name (in this case, the Cornwall Healthcare Trust). This in turn meant that the Admiral would have to reapply for his own job (in the sensible time-honoured way in which government departments do things!).[33] Initially he was the only nominee for the chairman's post of the new trust, but this was evidently not acceptable and 'the Minister asked for a choice of names[34] in accordance with (her) guidelines.' [Authors' proposed translation: 'including a woman who could then be chosen for the post'].

---

[31]The more perspicacious reader may discern a cause and effect relationship here!

[32]Manifestly some guidance was needed as to what was politically correct in these matters. Before the Admiral won his battle, your bewildered authors would have been unable to advise as they had been forced to the conclusion that it is quite acceptable to openly discriminate against people just so long as they happen to be middle-aged heterosexual, male, Anglo-Saxon and Church of England, i.e. the same as themselves.

[33]Mr Guy Pritchard, Sir Godfrey's learned counsel, described the Admiral's hard work in setting up the new amalgamated trust ironically as 'digging his own grave'.

[34]NHS Management Executive Committee guidelines also openly stated that; positive gender discrimination is allowed (they chose not to use the term *sexist* – see the Chapter 7 'Words That Are Not Very Nice'); they evidently point out that the magic word is opportunity.

A suitable lady was duly found (who like Virginia Bottomley was not only female but also a staunch supporter of the Conservative and Unionist Party) and duly appointed. Only two months later, however, the *Daily Telegraph* announced ADMIRAL WINS DAMAGES FOR SEX BIAS OVER HEALTH POST[xvii]. The article went on to state that the settlement came within hours of the resignation of Mrs X[35] and that earlier in the month 'the five non-executive directors passed an unprecedented vote of no confidence in her chairmanship.'

That was after less than three months! It was also reported there that Admiral Sir Godfrey had said that he did not want his job back. Of course he did not want to work in that shambles again – he was well out if it. All the Old Campaigner had ever wanted was to vindicate his good name and, more importantly, to expose the wrongdoers, to speak out for what is good and righteous, and to act as a champion for the downtrodden underdog, fighting a virtuous crusade against vulgar and irrational prejudice.

Clearly, even in these enlightened days, prejudice still lurks even at the highest level.

---

[35]Your authors have changed this name – she was not actually called Mrs X.

CHAPTER 4

DUTY, PRIVILEGE AND RESPONSIBILITY

Tippets At Derriford

Recently, the Royal Naval Hospital (RNH) Stonehouse in Plymouth was closed (along with all but one of the military hospitals in the United Kingdom). The unit became amalgamated with the NHS Derriford Hospital in that city and the Royal Naval Nurses now work there. They continue to wear their smart professional uniforms (maintained by themselves with much elaborate folding and starching) and are inordinately proud to do so. These uniforms include caps, and, during the winter, tippets![1] This is in contrast to the drab Jay Cloth-like outfits which the NHS Derriford nurses are supplied with. Much to the chagrin of the Nursing Stasi, patients at the hospital often complained when being looked after by the civilians, stating that they would rather be treated by one of the 'proper' nurses – i.e. one wearing a traditional nurse uniform. Some 'progressive' nurses might even

---

[1] The other group of people who wear red tippets are, of course, Her Majesty's Judges.

welcome the end of uniforms[2] – there is a strange feminist idea that the traditional uniform merely reinforces the role of the nurse as being somehow subservient to that of a doctor. Certainly, many nurses in administrative roles are quick to divest themselves of anything which might recall their origins, and specialist nurse practitioners who work in outpatients can be seen wearing their ordinary civilian clothes with a white coat – *just like a doctor.*[i]

It might well be that changes are not effected for such nefarious purposes and indeed it is far more likely that economy is the reason why nowadays nurses are dressed as cleaners. We found the following, which was fixed to the notice board in the Surgeons' Coffee Room in a District General Hospital, presumably by some frustrated surgeon who had found out that business tendering had compromised the quality of material provided.

It's unwise to pay too much, but it's worse to pay too little. When you pay too much you lose a little – that is all. When you pay too little, you sometimes lose everything because the thing you bought was incapable of doing the thing it was bought to do. The common law of business balance prohibits paying a little and getting a lot – it cannot be done. If you deal with the lowest bidder, it is well to add something for the risk you run and if you do that you will have enough to pay for something better.

John Ruskin 1819–1900

Impersonation
Readers may already have experienced that unreal Kafka-like

---

[2] Two of your authors have from time to time been lucky enough to meet with nurses who fall into this category (i.e. nurses who like to have their uniforms removed).

feeling – a sense of unreality – at some of the stories in this book. We do not blame you for your incredulity. It will be stretched to its very limits as the book unfolds. The next little cameo is unbelievable too, but the reader is assured of its veracity: the poor consultant in the tale is in the same club as one of your authors and the story is just as it was told to him. Suffice to say it concerns an ENT surgeon from Winchester.

On arrival at his usual outpatients clinic one morning, he was somewhat surprised to see a lady in a white coat with a stethoscope draped around her neck[3]. She somehow, despite this clever disguise, did not ring true. For a start, ENT surgeons don't usually use stethoscopes (until very recently, they had a circular mirror on a band around their head), secondly, she was carrying a clipboard with lots of papers clipped to it (and most doctors certainly do not carry clipboards). The plastic shoes were a bit of a give-away too.

Your authors' colleague, being reasonably quick on the uptake, smelled a rat and politely asked the intruder to identify herself.

'Oh I'm from audit', she replied indignantly.

'Please carry on with the clinic as though I'm not here!'

Had the reader not already perused the chapter on the Stasi, he might have reasonably assumed that even accountants would have known about confidentiality (after all, real chartered accountants are professionally bound not to divulge their clients' financial details). This lack of insight into how doctors work is, as

---

[3]This is usually taken to be the badge or regalia of a doctor in the late twentieth century. Our reader might be interested to know that from the fourteenth to seventeenth centuries this symbol would have been a glass flask containing urine. It appears that there are certain advantages to working in the twentieth century!

we have already touched upon, a great problem when non-qualified personnel are let into patient areas in hospitals. They don't really know how to behave (because this was not included in their course with their double-entry book-keeping) and so they continue to make the most awful gaffes.

When questioned further about her clever disguise, our hero was told dismissively that it should not worry him, and the auditor had merely worn these items 'to put the patients at their ease'.

Since most ENT surgeons are by nature tactful, diplomatic and unaggressive fellows (JRY is a Libran), he quietly told her to leave his clinic by the shortest possible route. A discreet veil will be drawn upon any suggestion as to where the stethoscope would be forcibly inserted if this advice were not immediately followed.

The reader may already feel that intrusion into the privacy of the consulting room and impersonation of a doctor are unbelievable enough stories. This, however, is only the beginning. When the surgeon had finished his first consultation of the day, having assumed this bad dream was now over, he then found that during this first patient's consultation, all his patients had been sent home by a senior Stasi, who now informed him that he had been suspended for his outrageous behaviour!

The Chairman of the Medical Executive Committee, however, called an emergency meeting of the Winchester hospital consultants who collectively demanded his immediate reinstatement. This was grudgingly done and the Chief Executive was instructed to write and apologise to all the patients who had been sent home. Money was then wasted by the Trust for them all to be seen again on an initiative basis (i.e. the Trust paid for them all to be seen privately by the same consultant at an 'out of hours' clinic). The female auditor was never charged with impersonating a doctor under the Medical Act 1858, and the

Winchester Trust can count itself very lucky that the story was not in the following day's tabloid newspapers.

Handmaidens of The Doctors[4]

The concept of nurses as handmaidens of the doctors is probably a hangover from the stereotypes portrayed on *Emergency Ward Ten* and *Doctor Kildare*[5], in which soppy staff nurses invariably drooled over clean-cut, handsome, healthy-looking housemen! Your authors strongly refute that this was ever the case in real-life[6]. It is certainly not the case nowadays. Nurses now are taking degrees in nursing and must be specialists in their own right. Some nurses are so professional that they are called 'nurse specialists'; yet others (presumably even more professional) are 'nursing consultants'. The reader should not be too surprised therefore to discover that there are even professors of nursing[7]. In some hospitals there are Professionally-Led (their choice of terminology, not ours) Clinical Service Teams (PLCSTs) in which the Nursing Stasi are so terribly professional that they act as the 'line-managers' for all sorts of people, including the librarian (who usually has a proper University degree) and even the hospital chaplain (we always thought that the chaplain's line manager was on a different net!).

In Sweden and the United States of America, there are even

---

[4]It was Thomas Carlyle (1795–1881) who in an Inaugural Address in Edinburgh in 1866 said, 'Maidservants, I hear people complaining, are getting instructed in the 'ologies'.

[5]Two television soap operas of the 1950s.

[6]To their knowledge, housemen have never looked clean-cut or wholesome!

[7]There are even chairs of chiropody and physiotherapy (Rao D S. Nurse Role Row Goes On. *Hospital Doctor* 15 January 1998, p25).

nurses who are anaesthetists and give anaesthetics quite successfully, but there are none who are *anesthesiologists*[8], who are all medically qualified and supervise nurse anaesthetists.

Some British consultants are happy about this and point out that a Swedish authority on the subject compared mortality figures in 1992 in Sweden with those in other Western countries, finding that 'anaesthesia was safest in Sweden where the nursing system prevails.'[ii] Notwithstanding this interesting comparison (which has been called into question on the grounds that the Swedes were a healthier and more robust ethnic group than most of the others anyway), quite a lot of consultant surgeons, including both your authors, would be more than willing to exchange their present anaesthetists for Swedish nurses, but believe it or not, this feeling is not universal. An ENT surgeon from Darlington was

> appalled to hear the suggestion that the solution to the shortage of anaesthetists was to train nurses to anaesthetise patients. When the inevitable disaster occurs, the consultant who still has overall responsibility for the care of the patient will be held to blame – not the nurse, the hospital or the Health Secretary. [iii]

We, and we would hope most of our colleagues[9], do not have any problem with the extended role of the nurse and hope it saves

---

[8]Your authors have not taken leave of their senses, nor are they trying to suck up to any American reader who might offer them a lucrative job; we simply use the American spelling because the word is only ever found there.

[9]The GMC's definition of a doctor's colleague is considered in greater detail later on – keep reading!

them all doing unnecessary work. They feel secure enough to know that none of these nursing 'specialists' or 'consultants' would ever put on white coats and sling stethoscopes around their necks and try to give the impression that they are doctors, which of course is in contravention of the Medical Act 1858. They are confident that if any patient mistook them, they would immediately disabuse them saying 'No! No! I am a nurse – not a doctor!'

Is this newly-found nurse independence a development marking the modern nurse graduate of the new millennium, or is it a return to the days when the doctor in the village cost too much and it was much cheaper if one felt ill to 'carry one's water to the wise woman'?[10] The cynic may well feel that the recent posts of nurse specialist are financially driven – a nurse's time is cheaper than that of a doctor.[11] The days when nursing was a practical job and the nurse did an apprenticeship (which unlike most apprenticeships was paid – albeit a pittance) are gone. The new era is that of the academic nurse, who will not be expected to make beds, hand out bedpans and wipe bottoms. The warm-hearted feminine lass (or lad) with a heart as big as a bucket (but who was totally non academic) now has no place as a nurse.[12] Talking to the 'grass-roots' nurses (still happily alive and well in most hospitals) on the wards, it would appear that the majority of experienced nurses are not at all happy with the changes that

---

[10] In *Twelfth Night* when his two friends feared Malvolio had gone mad, they sent a specimen of urine off to the uroscopist or water-caster who would diagnose, treat, and prognosticate on the appearance of the water alone.

[11] This does not mean of course that nurses are inferior, but just different.

[12] There is still an opening for them as Health Care Assistants of which there are two grades: HCA 2 and HCA 3 (which is senior). Your authors don't know what happened to HCA 1.

are taking place. They reckon that everything is becoming far too intellectual and say that if they were studious and learned, they would have gone into medicine instead.[13]

There are now (evidently serious) suggestions that all 'health care professionals' should complete the same basic years training. That is that chiropodists[14], doctors, ECG technicians, nurses, etc[15] should all attend the same basic foundation course! Remember that A-level requirements for medical students are amongst the highest for any profession. For them, the first year has traditionally been one of the most difficult academic hoops she[16] is ever made to jump through! Most doctors, however, would agree that it is not intellectual ability alone, but the facility to do dogged hard work, which is the principal quality which gets one through medical school. It is the skill to stay up all night and still retain the power to make decisions under stress which doctors in the past have always considered part of the job; nurses, remember, work shifts.

The first professional examinations have always been so arduous and demanding that they were used to sort out the sheep from the goats, since it was thought that to do this at the earliest stage seemed the best idea. Without wishing to seem too patronising to other health care professionals, we do wonder if student nurses and student chiropodists would welcome the same sort of gruelling examinations in anatomy, biochemistry and physiology.

---

[13]This does not, of course, mean that medicine is superior, but just different.

[14]Now called podiatrists.

[15]Here in alphabetical order.

[16]Since there are now more lady students than gentlemen, your authors have used the female pronoun.

Another option of course would be to follow suit with the rest of university training in the UK and 'dumb down' the basic medical science course. Your authors are confident that none of their readers would be so uncharitable as to suggest that perhaps things had gone just a teeny bit far. It was as long ago as 1577 that Harrison said in his *Description of Britain*: '*Tempora mutant, et nos mutamur in illis*'[17]. We must all change with the times. The whole of society has changed. Mascie-Taylor (a Stasi from a very respected family of proper scientists) averred in 1998 that: 'the doctor is different[18], the patient is different, and the medicine is different.'[iv]

At a day symposium 'NHS Day at the Royal Society of Medicine' held 8 July 1998, an eminent speaker summed up the paradox well by drawing attention to the fact that willing and efficient Medical Administrators are few and suspect to some colleagues; the new lay Managers are regarded as arrogant and interested in cost cutting and yet they are paid more than the consultants.[v] He goes on to say that:

> Today's consultants are undoubtedly more efficient than their predecessors and practising very good medicine in difficult circumstances. However, their place in the hierarchy is not at all what was envisaged in 1948.

The dignity of labour – a Victorian work ethic – has gone. It is now considered more dignified to be on the dole than work as a street cleaner or a lavatory attendant. People have no shame about

---

[17]Times change, and we are changed in them.

[18]Your authors do concede that the medicine and the patient are different, but as to the doctor, well the Stasi would like to think so.

being out of work (after all, it is not their fault, is it?). This same ethos (or lack of it) does not allow a young man to take up gainful employment as a shop assistant (considered in Victorian times a very good job); it is quite alright, however, for him to become a *trainee manager* at a shop[19]. In the past, young ladies found nothing degrading or debasing in being a handmaiden (indeed, some women rather enjoyed it).

One of your authors warmly remembers his first morning as a consultant. The sister-in-charge of the ENT ward had written to him to ask what time he would arrive at the hospital. She met him in the hospital lobby at half past eight prompt. After that she met him punctually there every Monday, Wednesday and Friday morning at half past eight prompt. As they walked together to the ward, she would brief him on any worries she had. After his ward round, she would take coffee with him in her office. After the formalities she would accompany him to the door of the ward.

One thing was very clear: she was neither his handmaiden, nor the handmaid to anyone else. Sister Jeffery was a professional nurse of the old school. Her patients were absolutely confident in her skills and felt safe and secure in her charge. She would not only expect her nurses to empty bedpans and wipe bottoms: she would help out herself if they were short staffed. She would expect the ward to be spotlessly clean, and expect her nurses to clean out cupboards and dust light fittings.[20] That was less than thirty years ago.

---

[19]The most amazing example of this was met by one of your authors whilst travelling by train from Leeds to Bradford. The ticket collector bore a badge bearing the title Revenue Protection Officer.

[20]With the advent of dangerous nosocomial bacteria such as methicillin resistant staphylococcus aureus (MRSA), nurses are once again starting to clean ward cupboards properly.

Nowadays when a consultant visits a ward other than the one on which he usually works (and perhaps where it is not generally known that he is a pernickety old dinosaur), it is not unusual for him to be told 'Mrs So-and-So is in such-and-such a bed in bay 4'. He is then presumably expected to go to that bed unaccompanied and get on with it. The correct procedure, of course, is to politely ask the nurse if she would be so kind as to accompany one. On such occasions, they often look quite surprised to have been asked. If this is not done, then any decisions that are made at the bedside will not be properly communicated; the nursing staff will not know about them; valuable time (of both doctor and nurse) will be wasted; and what ought to be done will inevitably remain undone. Verbal instructions are always better understood, and if they are accompanied by written directives, one may be sure that they will be properly executed.

One should, of course, be charitable and blame this reluctance of nurses to accompany the doctor on the ward on the shortage of nursing staff, which has been caused by the Stasi.

One of us had the great privilege to once work with Professor Pierre Durel, the foremost venereologist in Paris. The old professor told some wonderful stories of how he used to work as Babinski's[21] houseman at the Salpetrière in Paris, where the *chef d'infirmières*[22] would carry a towel and a silver bowl of warm water to wash the patients before Babinski examined the soles[23]

---

[21]Joseph Francois Felix Babinski (1857–1932). One of the 'Fathers' of neurology.

[22]Matron.

[23]Babinski's test is a famous and useful test in neurology in which the sole of the foot is stroked with a metal instrument. If the toes go up instead of down, this is very significant. (Babinski J F F. *Comptes rendues hebdomadaires des séances de la Société de Biologie*, Paris 1896; 3:207.

of their feet. One cannot help but wonder if the present day 'chip-on-the-shoulder' Nursing Stasi would expect the great old man to carry his own towel and bowl. One got the impression that he would not have minded in the least,[24] but the matron would have had an apoplexy at the very thought.[25] It might be considered that she was acting as a handmaiden to the great man, but she never lost any dignity in washing feet. Indeed, she was following a very illustrious example.[26]

The following – part of an interview[vi] with Sam Norman, daughter of the film critic Barry Norman – is revealing about the public perception of nurses; she went on to marry a doctor.

> When I was about six I told my dad that I'd like to be a nurse. He said: 'Oh no, you don't. If you're going to be anything, be a doctor. Aim high and if you hit anywhere in the middle, it won't be too bad.'

It is not just from the general public – the *BMA News Review* recently carried a piece entitled 'Nurse to Doctor Medical Upgrade' in which a 27 year-old doctor describes how she

> ... realised she was capable of a lot more ... I started nurse

---

[24]Professor Durel told another story that Babinski went home precipitantly in the middle of one ward round, when the matron told him that his wife's soufflé was nearing perfection. Babinski was over 6 ft tall and loved his food.

[25]Which, of course, Babinski would have been eminently able to diagnose!

[26]'Jesus... laid aside his garments; and took a towel and girded himself. After that he poureth water into a basin, and began to wash the disciples' feet, and to wipe them with the towel wherewith he was girded.' (Gospel according to St John Ch 13 3-5) – gird means to wrap around like a girdle.

training when I was 17. I was soon very frustrated with the job. It was not enough for me just to do basic nursing tasks. I wanted to know about anatomy, physiology and basic pathology.[vii]

Your authors wager that that did not endear her to her former nursing teachers! It will probably come as no surprise that the transition from nurse to doctor was made harder because some of her former colleagues branded her a deserter – as she puts it:

I had no problems from doctors but I had problems from nurses. Some of them were very supportive and thought it was great but some of them could not understand why I was doing it. They had the attitude that 'oh, you don't want to be one of us'.

Can I Take A Verbal Order, Doctor?

Nursing and medicine have always shared a close and intimate relationship.[27] We have always admired the professionalism and dedication of nurses. Their devotion and endless care to patients act as a shining example to us all. This duty to their patients, however, is not mirrored by a similar loyalty and commitment to each other. Doctors have been criticised in the past (sometimes justifiably), if not for actively covering up for their colleagues, at least for the 'Cloak of Silence' when one of their number has gone astray. Nurses do not show this loyalty to other nurses, however. If a nurse is ever accused of some minor misdemeanour, she can

---

[27]Some readers, who may have played Doctors and Nurses as children (or even older) might think this should read Doctors and Nurses have always shared a close and intimate relationship. Sadly, your authors refute this.

forget any idea of Pankhurstian shoulder to shoulder[28] sisterliness; she is more likely to be the victim of a bitchy witch-hunt, and find herself pilloried by her colleagues. Your authors would strongly like to refute any sexist suggestion that this is because women are bitchier than men – some male nurses can be real bitches!

The sad story of Sister Pat Cooksley, a well-respected ward sister of thirty-seven years nursing experience underlines the lack of solidarity and sorority that a nurse in need can expect. In May 1994 Sister Pat was summoned to work at seven in the morning to be told that she had been suspended. She was told that she must not speak to anyone in the hospital and escorted unceremoniously from the premises by a security guard. We have spoken to senior consultants at Derriford Hospital, Plymouth where this shabby little event took place to see if, as they had suspected, there was any hidden agenda behind her suspension. We were not surprised to learn that Sister Pat was the wife of a specialist at the hospital. A consultant described her as:

> An old-fashioned, highly intelligent, really high-quality ward sister, who was absolutely streets ahead of any of the new nurse managers in the hospital. She didn't want to be a ward manager.[viii]

She did not wish to change her nursing practices to the financial ethos of the new NHS. She appeared brighter than the Stasi and her main motives in life were not driven by money: she was therefore seen as a threat. She had evidently already spoken out

---

[28]The battle song of the suffragettes was called 'Shoulder to Shoulder'. Another suffragette slogan, believe it or not, was 'Down with the Trousers'!

against the Trust when she had thought that patients would suffer because of financial cutbacks.[ix] She must be got[29] rid of.

The manner of her suspension was as follows: a charge of gross professional misconduct was brought against her after she failed to obtain a doctor's signature[30] on a repeat prescription which had been authorised by telephone.[x]

There had been a two-month gap between the alleged incident and her dismissal. She herself was stunned. On the day of her sacking, a nurse on the neurosurgical ward (she has asked that her name is not disclosed, because she is fearful of reprisals) said that she was 'devastated' and that Sister Cooksley was 'one of the best and most hard-working nurses'.[xi] A nursing auxiliary on the same ward also said: 'Sister Cooksley is one of the most dedicated nurses I have ever had the pleasure to meet. The patients love her, and so do her staff.'[xii]

'Where is the lack of support from nursing colleagues?' our discriminating reader may well by now be asking. The above two anonymous reports were the immediate reactions at the time of the suspension by her own colleagues.

But things were going to change.

Soon enough, the screw began to turn. Would it be uncharitable to think that after a couple of weeks, nurses had been knobbled – that they had been 'got at' by the Stasi when the headline SACKING OF NURSE BACKED BY 25 SISTERS appeared in the same newspaper[xiii]? Your authors have always had a cynical nature, and it is their opinion that pressure was being brought to

---

[29]US 'gotten.'

[30]Standing Operational Procedures in place there demand that these be counter-signed by the prescribing doctor within 24 hours.

bear on other nurses pointing out on which side their bread was buttered. Sisterly support was dwindling like snow before the springtime sun. As more and more sycophantic gutless nurses came out of the Derriford Hospital woodwork, poor Sister Pat was getting less and less backing from her colleagues.

Then something totally unexpected took place. Overnight, an amazing amount of support appeared from an unforeseen source. Owing to national media coverage there was a public outcry. A march was organised. Relatives of patients, and patients themselves picketed the hospital protesting against Pat Cooksley's suspension. A foolhardy Stasi tried to stop the marchers, but was lucky not to be trampled underfoot by the demonstrators. They descended on the hospital (some in wheelchairs) carrying banners with the slogans WE TRUST SISTER PAT and WE DISTRUST THE TRUST. One read TREACHEROUS, RUTHLESS, UNJUST, SECRETIVE, TYRANNICAL – the first letters highlighted to spell TRUST.[xiv]

The pathetic response of the Trust was to persuade sixty of Pat's colleagues to write to the Health Minister Virginia Bottomley supporting the Trust's decision. This magnanimous act was then leaked to the local newspaper.

But senior consultants and junior doctors backed Sister Cooksley in her fight to be reinstated.[xv] The Trust Chairman capitulated and gave in to public pressure and she was reinstated in January 1995. One feature of this whole sad case is very clear. It was not Sister Cooksley's nursing colleagues who had rallied around her in her hour of need. Nursing Stasi had pushed Pat out of the hospital in the same way an overgrown cuckoo ousts the rightful chick from its nest. As time went on, more and more nurses joined in to support the Stasi in their witch-hunt against her. Even in the face of overwhelming public opinion and when the hospital medical staff supported Pat, her colleagues were apparently bent on crucifying her. Did these treacherous nurses at Derriford turn their backs on Sister Cooksley because there were fearful that they might lose their own jobs if they did not toe the line? Nurses hardly ever seemed to support each other, and the turncoat nurses knew that. It is always easier to pick off individuals. Were they frightened to support her, because it had been suggested that it might be their turn next?

Spite And Malice In South Molton

One nurse was not quite so lucky. South Molton is a small market town in North Devon. Carol Rudd married a local farmer and started to work there as a health visitor in 1975, and soon became a popular and well-respected member of the community. A local businessman said: 'Carol was exactly what you would want of a health visitor to be – practical, sensible and efficient.'[31]

In 1986, however, as a result of a reorganisation, former administrator, Allwyn McKibbin, with no experience of health visiting was given a job in a South Molton Health Centre, working alongside Carol. The two women never hit it off. Allwyn soon criticised Carol's 'minimalist approach to note-keeping'; in turn, Carol was unimpressed by Allwyn's passion for filing.[xvi] Dear reader, you would be forgiven if you consider that what happened three years later was a malicious and spiteful vendetta by a health authority against a farmer's wife. It seems once again that one does not necessarily have to be a doctor to fall prey to the Stasi's incomparable incompetence and malice. Mrs Rudd's story is an example of how public funds can be wasted recklessly when a point is to be scored.

The initial offensive against Carol Rudd was launched in June

---

[31]This was quoted in *The Sunday Times* 22 February 1998.

1989, when a charge of gross incompetence was levelled against her by Allwyn McKibbin. As no evidence could be found to support this allegation, it had to be dropped. Three months later, in September, the authority began, in the words of *The Sunday Times* 'its persecution of the midwife which would last for eight years'. As we later show in the chapter on disciplining of doctors (and it is a well-known principle in many organisations), the next move in such a battle is to check up on all claims for reimbursement. Travel claims dating back many years are trawled for some discrepancy. The authority proceeded to do this – but could find nothing wrong. What happened next is described by Carol as 'like something out of a bad novel'.

The authority sent three nursing Stasi to undertake a covert surveillance by following her on her rounds (even taking long-range photographs!). This occurred for a period of four weeks (evidently over a slack period for nursing managing!) during September 1995. When she submitted her travel claim for that month they mounted a dawn raid[32] and removed files, personal papers and even the contents of her wastepaper basket! Let us be quite clear who these people were, or rather who they were not. They were not policemen with properly authorised warrants – they were work colleagues looking for dirt. A further seven months then elapsed. It can only be assumed that further sophisticated high level investigative work was going on. Carol, on the other hand, was dismissed on charges of 'not visiting patients and filing false mileage expenses totalling £34.18.'

It was not for a further four years, in 1993, that a hearing took

---

[32]For our non-military readers, this means an attack which takes place at dawn – ie very early in the morning. The authors are willing to bet that the personnel in question (unlike soldiers) either worked a night shift or got a day off later 'in lieu'.

place. What transpired is simply incredible, and would not be out of place in Kafka's *The Trial*. It is difficult to believe that these events did not occur in some police state. Carol's patients had been approached by the Stasi (former nurses), who had knocked on doors in the South Molton area masquerading as researchers on a regional survey. They asked what each patient thought of Carol's performance. When the truth eventually emerged (at a UKCC hearing against the three nurse mangers) the furious patients claimed that not only had their testimonies been obtained dishonestly, but had been twisted out of context, and in some cases fabricated. The patients were actually very supportive of Nurse Rudd and found her to be very competent.

In contrast, the incompetence of the authority in their illegal persecution of one of their staff beggars belief. At Carol's own hearing it emerged that those employed to follow her had knocked off from work at 5.30 pm (your authors are frankly amazed that they stayed so long!). It came out at the hearing that Carol (who was not a 9 to 5 manager type) had continued working until she had completed all her calls, even when it meant working well into the evening. The whole case against her collapsed when it became obvious that her spies had only followed her for a part of her work. On the day 'when they did manage to keep up with her, the mileage counts tallied'. Sadly, the enquiry never did ascertain whether they thought nobody ever worked past 5.30, or whether they were damned if *they* were going to!

The UKCC ruled that Carol Rudd was cleared of any fraud or dishonesty and that she should return to work. The North Devon Authority did not give her her job back, however, and *The Sunday Times* announced in February 1998 that at least £200,000 had already been spent in legal fees (as well as untold hours of fruitless work) by it trying to regain the £34. It had forecast a £25 million budget deficit, though. Nor did the authority pay her the expense claim for September 1989, which was still outstanding. To your authors' best knowledge, she was never reinstated, nor was this claim for travel expenses honoured.

Top Doc Bugged[33]

In the late 1970s the new Royal Liverpool Hospital was opened. The old Royal was a beautiful and much-loved Victorian Gothick building. It had an impressive entrance hall from which wide corridors lined by attractive wall-tiles led off to a number of old but practical Nightingale wards. The Liverpudlians loved it – in contrast to the stark new building which replaced it, the architecture of which might best be described as 'late Soviet municipal'. The eyesore was only a few hundred yards away from the lovely old building, and one of the features of which it proudly boasted before it opened was that all the lifts[34] in the building would have emergency telephones. Only a week after the People's Palace of Medicine opened, however, none of these phones remained in the lifts, but many houses in Liverpool now had a bedside telephone!

One might reasonably expect that the phones in the consultants' offices would not be tampered with; one might further hope (principally because of the absolute need for patient confidentiality) that the telephone in the consultant's office would be a secure line. An amazing tale told to us by a colleague[35]

---

[33]No, dear reader, your authors have not lost all their literary style – this was the headline in the local newspaper.

[34]US: 'elevators'.

[35]We use the word in its officially approved GMC manner.

at the Luton and Dunstable Hospital shows that this is clearly *not* the case.

The saga involves a progressive young radiologist by the name of Dr John Spencer, who according to other consultants in the hospital had made 'very significant improvements' to the X-ray department.[xvii] Among other developments, he had been instrumental in the acquisition of a brand new MRI scanner, which had been installed only a few weeks before his annual holiday. He was looking forward to using this wonderful new bit of kit, but on his return, he noticed one or two things which were not quite right. When he arrived in his office, the first little abnormality was that all his personal mail, received during his holiday, had been opened. Although this had not been done before, and is technically unlawful,[36] he did not take it too much to heart. Your authors are both quite pleased if their hospital mail is opened and dealt with during their absence, because this will reduce their burden on return. They don't however expect letters marked 'confidential' or even 'personal' to be opened. Not only had all Dr Spencer's mail been opened during his absence but each letter and circular had been rubber-stamped by the office of the Chief Executive of the Trust!

The next anomaly, which irritated him was that his computer, which had been working well when he left, was now 'on the blink'. Both your authors are surgeons whose ability to use computers is marginally better than that of a tortoise! But Dr Spencer is used to pushing buttons on sophisticated X-ray machines and, after a cursory investigation, soon found an extra cable at the back. This

---

[36]In law, an offence against the Post Office Act which requires that mail should be delivered to the addressee only and not tampered with except by the Post Office itself when returning undelivered or undeliverable mail.

was, would you believe it, leading to his telephone. He unplugged this cable and left his office to visit the adjacent WC. Whilst there, he happened to notice some new ducting coming through the wall from his office and leading to a box.[37] Being not only inquisitive but practical, he soon had the casing off to find a tape-recorder bearing the admonition 'Do not disturb' inside. He traced the wires back to the telephone on his desk and ascertained that this bugging device was activated by the use of his telephone!

The BMA never ceases to be a tower of strength and source of invaluable advice at times like these. He contacted them (on a different telephone!) – and was told to report the matter to the police. When the police arrived, they were very interested in the unlawful telephone tapping device.[38] They wanted to take it back with them to the police station. However, they were not going to touch anything, which said 'Do not disturb' without permission. When they tried to get this authority from the Chief Executive, she could not be found. So they left! We quote from Peter Bruggen: No real sense of clarity was achieved until the last two minutes of the day[39], when the telephone rang.[xviii]

It was the Chief Executive, a woman who according to other consultants at the hospital had an 'extremely aggressive' style of management[xix.] She had rung to tell him that he was suspended!

The series of events following this are even more bewildering. One of the first positive moves by management came from the

---

[37]For a full version the reader is directed to Chapter 17, 'What You Learn When You Take A Pee in Peter Bruggen's excellent book *Who Cares?* (1997).

[38]Article 8 of the European Convention of Human Rights states: 'There shall be no interference by a public authority except such as in accordance with law'.

[39]Your authors are surprised she had not gone home some hours before this.

Trust Chairman (who, prior to coming to work at the hospital had worked in the motor industry). He burned the tape!

A second amazing revelation was the alarming disclosure of the installing engineer of the bugging device; he claimed that this was a regular feature of his work in NHS hospitals! Perhaps the most disturbing feature of the whole disgraceful saga is the cloak of secrecy which then descended. Only a few facts are now clear. Dr Spencer remained suspended until 'a negotiated deal' was reached. This usually means a hefty financial settlement is given to the victim (particularly if he is younger than fifty). In these negotiated deals it is customary to impose a confidentiality agreement on the doctor. This 'gagging clause' ensures that the public never finds out just how much of its money has been wasted. Understandably, poor Dr Spencer was severely distressed by the whole sorry episode. He had lost his job and his career; his health was affected. As at least one newspaper reported, his silence, however, had been effectively bought and he will now say nothing about the phone-tapping incident. The Stasi have committed a series of, at worst, unlawful and, at best, dishonourable acts. They opened his mail; they tapped his telephone without the authority of the Home Office; they destroyed evidence required by the police by burning the audiotape; they suspended him without reference to the GMC or the courts; they damaged his health and destroyed his career. Yet what did he ever do wrong? Perhaps because of the clandestine stealth with which it was dealt and the underhand concealment with which his silence was bought, we shall never know.[40]

---

[40]Your authors were going to call this section 'None shall utter her secret' (borrowed from *Alma Mater* by Sir Arthur Quiller-Couch) but thought that the banner headline 'Top Doc Bugged' was a bit more punchy!

Whatever it was, it cannot have been that terrible because the GMC or police were not involved.

Under the same veil of furtiveness, the Chief Executive and Personnel Officer were suspended, but the Trust Chairman who had burned the tape was not. The Chief Executive was later reinstated but shortly afterwards, with increasing pressure this 'exceptional chief executive' who had been 'totally trustworthy and a first class employee', resigned.

One of your authors has a pal who is a consultant gynaecologist at that hospital and he certainly had a good laugh at this description. Neither he nor any of the other consultants there have ever found out what the so-called misdemeanour of their former colleague was.

No one can make his or her own informed judgement, because nobody knows the facts. And Dr John Spencer is not going to tell us – if he did he would break his contract and lose his pension.

CHAPTER 5

FEES AND
REMUNERATION

Not by Bread Alone[1]

Medical fees constitute an index of the training of the profession at any given period, and of the standing of its members. It was Osler's own idea that volumes of his recorded fees should be preserved for their probable interest to posterity.[2] It perhaps reflects well on the profession as a whole that despite the presence of waiting lists (not yet incorporated into literature as a British phenomenon as typical as warm beer, seaside landladies, etc) there is a remarkable scarcity of scandal regarding bribes, 'baksheesh', 'blat' or anything else used in other countries to enable the ordinary citizen to oil the wheels of a state organization to his advantage. Nevertheless, great writers such as George Bernard Shaw long ago sounded the warning:

If you are going to have doctors you had better have doctors

---

[1] Matthew IV, verse 4 tells us that: 'Man shall not live by bread alone, but every word that proceedeth out of the mouth of God.'

[2] William Osler, one of the giants of the twentieth century medical world.

well off; just as if you are going to have a landlord you had better have a rich landlord. Taking all the round of professions and occupations, you will find that every man is the worse for being poor; and the doctor is a specially dangerous man when poor.[i]

He also drew attention to the thorny problem of 'you pay for what you (don't) get':

There would never be any public agreement among doctors if they did not agree on the main point of the doctor always being in the right. Yet the two guinea man never thinks that the five shilling man is right; if he did, he would be understood as confessing to an overcharge of £1:17s. Thus even the layman has to be taught that infallibility is not quite infallible, because there are two qualities of it to be had at two prices.[ii]

Cynicism can often be found when dealing with the remuneration of the medical profession, as this extract from Elizabeth Gaskell's *Wives and Daughters* reveals:

Mr. Gibson used to tell him that his motto would always be 'Kill or cure,' and to this Mr. Coxe once made answer that he thought is was the best motto a doctor could have; for if he could not cure the patient, it was surely best to get him out of his misery quietly, and at once. Mr. Wynne looked up in surprise, and observed that he should be afraid that such putting out of misery might be looked upon as homicide by some people. Mr. Gibson said in a dry tone, that for his part he should not mind the imputation of homicide, but that it would not do to make away with profitable patients in so speedy a manner; and that he thought that as long as they were willing and able to pay two-and-sixpence for the doctor's visit, it was his duty to keep them alive; of course when they became paupers the case was different.[3]

Of course, everything is relative. J G Ballard always said that before writing *Empire of the Sun* he earned about as much as an English G.P.; and after Spielberg made the movie he earned about as much as an American G.P.[4]

There is a feeling, which the authors (erroneously) thought was confined to the lay public, that medicine was a calling which had reward enough in itself. Any further remuneration was superfluous. What nonsense! This is the worst form of snobbery (as all the best people agree) but we agree that there has been a certain medical disdain for written contracts. This can have many repercussions of which we are sure the reader knows many, perhaps even personal, examples. The following extract from a novel published in 1969 refers to the growing cynicism of doctors and their role as state employees[iii]:

'We've been done, that's what,' he said savagely. 'Done. We went into the bloody scheme under certain conditions and now the bloody conditions aren't being kept.'
  'Yes, they are,' I said.
  'They're not.'
  'Course they are, Harry,' I said soothingly. 'You're a little bit potty today, that's all.'

[3]Quoted in Klass P. *A Not Entirely Benign Procedure*. New York: Putman, 1987, p.91.

[4]Quoted by Will Self. *The Cost of Letters*. Brentford: Waterstones, 1998, p.126.

'What do you know about it? They promised us so much money and they're not paying up and they won't.'

'Harry,' I said. 'Be reasonable. You've got a contract so all you have to do is sue. You've heard of suing, it's for breach of contract.'

'There's no contract.'

I clicked my tongue. 'Must be. You haven't looked.'

'Don't keep telling me I haven't looked,' he shrieked, 'I have. Everybody has. All they said was we'd be all right, they were honest men, they'd fix it up after we joined.'

I laughed. 'And they didn't'.

'They didn't. You've got it. You're bright this afternoon; sharp as a bloody razor.'

'Very trying for you, Harry,' I said. 'but let's not place the blame on the Government boys. They never do what they promise, it's a rule. This is embodied by implication in the constitution. You have to have an enforceable contract, and naturally I assumed you had one.'

'That's easy to say now,' he said, calming down. 'But you'd have believed them at the time.'

I smiled and shook my head.

'Look, John, a fellow looks at you with candid eyes and says: "I promise you this, my record says I'm responsible, I promise." Naturally you believe him.'

'With candid eyes?' I said. 'Be your age.'

'Then when you turn round it's some other bastard and he says he can't be held responsible for his predecessor. By then it's too late.'

The Accursed Power that Stands on Privilege[5]

Enoch Powell is a name that is more often associated with immigration, but during his incumbency as Minister of Health he made an (unusually) incorrect statement about emigration. He stated that there was categorically 'no emigration of doctors'. He said this in the early sixties during the so-called 'Brain Drain'. A professor of medicine, who was very concerned about doctors leaving the UK in their droves, asked the Minister to clarify how he could be so very certain about this assertion. Mr. Powell said he had looked at the number of doctors state pension funds, and that there had been no decline in this number; the conclusion must be therefore that doctors were not emigrating. The truth of the matter was very different however. Initial perusal showed that the number of funds indeed had not declined but more detailed scrutiny showed that quite a large number had not received any recent contributions. What in fact had happened was that doctors were emigrating, but they had forgotten to reclaim their pension contributions – either because doctors are not financially motivated or because dreams of the fortune they were about to make in America had driven it out of their heads. Clearly the emigrés had never heard of the old adage[6] about looking after the pennies.

Doctors quite often cannot be bothered to claim their travel expenses back. This is a recurrent problem and causes much concern amongst the accountants and pencil-pushers, who often develop an obsession about it. Quite frankly, there are usually more important things to be dealt with in the hospital

---

[5]Hillaire Belloc: *Epigrams on a General Election*.

[6]Eighteenth century proverb.

consultant's life than filling out even more forms, the effort of which is rarely worth the candle. A consultant in East Anglia created an important precedent in this matter, though. He sent off his monthly travel claims in one large batch – for the previous six years! Somewhat predictably, the dullards in 'accounts' sent a very sniffy reply saying something along the lines that they couldn't possibly countenance paying anything more than the previous month's claim and that it was clearly stated on the forms. What the sparkling wits at Wages and Salaries had not reckoned on, however, was that this particular consultant was doubly qualified, with degrees in both medicine and the law. He took the case to law – and won back his six years of travel expenses. The judgement was that legitimate travel claims are a *right* and not some *privilege* to be handed out by the largesse of some finance director. Like any other debt, they have to be submitted within seven years.

If any reader has any similar difficulty, the threat to sue for the claim under the Small Claims Court of the County Court is usually sufficient. Your authors, it may not surprise the reader to learn, are no novices in this field. When the hospital finance department wrote a rather high-handed and somewhat disrespectful letter to all consultants advising them that any travel claim later than three months would not be paid, one of your authors responded by sending Small Claim Court application forms (which he had collected from the County Court) to all his colleagues. He included a covering letter advising them how to apply and pointing out that the small court handling fee should be charged to the Director of Finance.[iv]

This did nothing to enhance the warm relationship he had always striven to preserve between himself and the Stasi. The Director of Personnel wrote back to him:

I believe that Trust's is being reasonable, and that it would be unwise for anyone to rely on the precedents to which you refer.[v]

We reproduce the reply with the original dodgy use of English so typical of the Stasi (to which we have referred elsewhere) uncorrected. The use of the word 'reasonable' ten times in a four-paragraph letter certainly stresses the point at issue (and after all we all know just how reasonable the Trust's).

An intelligent (dare one say reasonable?) observer with a rudimentary knowledge of economics might be forgiven for thinking that the Trust would have welcomed late travel reimbursement claims (particularly so if they were a year or two late!). That way, the gold in the Trust's coffers could be accruing interest on the unclaimed money. This is however not the case.

It is all a matter of budgets! The whole of the hospital income and expenditure is compartmentalized into a series of budgets, and the dull, narrow-minded hospital finance departments have no intention of letting money from one year's consultants' travel claim pigeon-hole get into another. Perhaps this would be an appropriate place to mention the important relationship between intelligence and flexibility. The interested reader should consult J P Guilford's *The Nature of Human Intelligence* that points out that versatility, flexibility and creativity are the essence of intelligence.

Imagine standing at a bus stop waiting for a bus to arrive: you see the correct bus coming down the road towards you, and then you feel in your left hand jacket pocket for your bus fare. Then, horror upon horror, you find that that pocket (your bus fare pocket) is empty. Luckily your right hand trouser pocket has a couple of quid in it. But you cannot use that – that is only for taxis! You quickly look down the road to the taxi rank and it is empty. But you cannot spend taxi money on a bus journey – that is a different budget! So, you walk down to the empty taxi rank, wait for a taxi, and spend much more on the same journey.

That is the logic which the NHS finance departments use. If housewives were to behave in the same way, then half the children in the country would probably never get fed. But then again, the average housewife can manipulate budgets, organise problems according to priority, handle several crises that occur at the same time and manage the daily work time with far greater ease than these so-called 'managers'.

Perks of the Job

There always have been 'perks of the job', as is shown by the letter written in Vienna by Sigmund Freud to Martha Bernays, 16 Jan 1885:

> ....takes the liberty of asking if and when the Herr Hofrat can be seen on an important personal matter. The usual crowd, usual anxious whispering among the people around me, whether I was a doctor and would be admitted before them who had already been waiting for so long.

More recently, an outcry ensued when a hospital in Aberdeen announced that its members of staff would be accelerated (for those devotees of the newspeak this would probably read as 'fast-tracked') up the waiting list as the smooth running of the hospital was being compromised by sickness amongst its workers. It is a principle not unknown to both industry and the trade unions. It was stopped owing to overwhelming political and public pressure. The benefit of private health insurance or preferential treatment is thought to be unacceptable for those working in the health service – presumably because then their striving to make it work might be compromised. In other words the perceived wisdom is that workers in the NHS only work hard to ensure that standards are acceptable should they themselves require them. A politician's stance has been that doctors should be rewarded but that the state should get something in return, Aneurin Bevan holding that:

> I cannot dispense with the principle that the payment of a doctor must in some degree be a reward for zeal, and there must be some degree of punishment for lack of it.

Of course, he was not treading any new ground, though it is a moot point as to whether he would have had the courage to put forward such views before a group of, for example, South Wales miners. He was simply taking Charles Darwin's dictum of 'the big differences between individuals are not in their abilities but in their willingness to work' a step further. Not all doctors are driven by sheer avarice, though historical examples of beneficence do not perhaps make as good reading. One example which underlines the idea that there is no pleasing some people is that of Edward Long Fox. He completed his medical training in 1781 and joined his father Joseph in practice in Falmouth. Joseph ran a sideline in merchant shipping, and in the fighting with France, could have received £22,000 – his share of the loot plundered from enemy vessels. On principle (he was a Quaker), he gave it all back apart from £120 which went unclaimed. Edward volunteered to go to France to try to return it, precipitating Falmouth's local newspaper to cynically and sarcastically write that apart from the nation's enemies, only his patients would applaud his trip: while he was away they could expect to enjoy good health!

Geoffrey Chaucer in the *Canterbury Tales* tells us how much his Doctour of Physick was fond of gold. He tells us:

> For gold in physick is a cordiall[7]
> Therefore he lovede gold in especial.[vi]

Chaucer did not say that he was in any way mercenary, but that he was partial to gold because it was good medicine (aurum potabile, drinkable gold – used not for arthritis but for heartburn) and we are left to draw our own conclusions.

John Arderne (1307–1390), an English surgeon who wrote the definitive contemporary treatise on anal fistulae tells us of the fourteenth century way of paying the surgeon which was evidently three-fold: an initial fee, then an annuity for life, and in addition one or more suits of clothes (liveries) yearly. Arderne writes:

> Ask of a great man an hundred marks or £40 with robes and a fee of an hundred shillings (£5) yearly for life. Of less men[8] let him ask £40 or 40 marks without further fees; and let him take not less than an hundred shillings for never in all my life took I less than an hundred shillings.

Hammond (an American) writing in 1960 considered this fee 'stupendous even for *a worthi man and a gret*,' and translated them into $3,500–$4,000 'modern American currency'.[vii]

The practice of an annuity certainly lingered until the end of

---

[7]'Cordiall' was a heart stimulant from *cordis*, Latin: heart.

[8]The annual income of a fourteenth-century labourer was £4.

the seventeenth century.[viii] Shakespeare mentions the physician's fee in *Pericles*:

> Thy sacred physic shall receive such pay,
> As thy desires can wish.[ix]

He does not however say exactly how much the fee is. D'Arcy Power investigated the question in a 1909 paper entitled 'The Fees of Our Ancestors'. He finds that during the seventeenth century the 'noble' (later to become the 'angel' and each worth between 6 shillings and 8 pence and 10 shillings) was the customary fee. This was raised to 21 shillings at the Restoration[x] with the introduction of the new guinea coin.[9] Although the guinea coin was discontinued in 1813, it was still used for many years by doctors, barristers and horse-dealers and sometimes by art-dealers and tailors.[xi]

Pecunia Non Olet[10]

Apparently very few laymen are aware what an NHS consultant's salary is, and, of course the whole issue is further blurred with false concepts about how much money they earn in private practice. We continue to be surprised at just how little idea the general public have with respect to private consultation fees

---

[9] Sir Robert Holmes in 1666 captured 160 Dutch vessels in Schelling Bay containing lots of gold bullion from Cape Coast Castle in Guinea. This rich prize was coined into gold pieces each stamped with an elephant, Africa and called 'guineas' to commemorate the valuable capture.

[10] 'Money does not smell.' The origin of this comes from Vespasian's reply to Titus, who objected to a tax on public lavatories in Ancient Rome; he held a coin under Titus's nose and asked if it smelled; when he was told it didn't he replied '*Atque e lotio est*' ('And it is made from urine!').

(they appear to think that either they are very cheap or extortionately expensive, but seldom give the impression that they are reasonable). Having said that, most patients are aware that nowadays there is only one payment (per item of service) and that an annuity is no longer expected. Nor do we get suits of clothes. One has to admit to an occasional unexpected and unsolicited bottle of wine, but neither of your authors have ever (to date) received a livery!

There is an apocryphal story of how the initial figure for a consultant's salary was arrived upon when the NHS was being set up in 1946. There was evidently a meeting in the Houses of Parliament between Aneurin Bevan and 'Corkscrew Charlie' (Lord Charles Moran, President of the Royal College of Physicians, and Private Physician to Sir Winston Churchill). The Minister of Health asked Lord Moran what he thought would be 'about the right amount' and Corkscrew Charlie tore up a cigarette packet (Presidents of the RCP evidently used to smoke in those days!) and scribbled a few quick calculations down on the back of it. Bevan took it away and later used it in the calculation of a consultant's salary.[11]

The amount implicitly assumed that the hospital specialist would also undertake some managerial duties as an everyday part of his job; there was nobody else to do it in those days anyway. The rules were written then before the Revolution when consultants just got on with administration as a matter of course. Nowadays, however, the consultant is faced with a dilemma. One is now placed in a schizophrenic situation in which a witless Stasi has been unnecessarily added to the equation. The consultant

---

[11]The more official version is that it was decided by the Spens Committee (of which Lord Moran was a member) – see Rivett G. *Cradle to Grave*. 1998, p.88.

knows that these supernumeraries are paying themselves extremely large sums of money. Most members of the public are totally unaware (and often horrified to learn) that the *starting* salary of a chief executive is much more that the *highest* rate NHS salary for a consultant at the top of his pay scale. Because the consultant is well aware of this, however, he is placed in what the Americans call a 'no-win situation'. He knows that the so-called managers would be totally unable to run the place on their own, because they don't have any understanding of how a hospital works. If, therefore, the specialist gets on with his job (as he always has done) he will be doing the Stasi's job for them – and perpetuating the post-Revolution myth that they have some role to play. The alternative, however, to leave it to the so-called managers means that nothing ever gets done. In practice the line of least resistance is usually followed and the consultant continues to do the administration so that the wheels of the hospital keep turning.

It has always been expected that the consultants would supplement their NHS salaries with large fees from private practice. Indeed, one of your authors knew of a consultant plastic surgeon in South Manchester who was a fully paid-up and unashamed member of the British Communist Party and who avowed he had no problems with his conscience when he charged large private fees for this very reason.

Some consultants choose not to have a private practice (usually for personal, political or ethical reasons) and indeed private practice is rare in some parts of Scotland. In the past, professors working in medical schools were certainly not allowed to have any income from private earnings. They could take on private cases, but the fees had to go into the rigorously regulated medical school coffers. Obviously in certain regions it was not too difficult to make a small fortune by milking the private practice, and it was understandably often suggested (sometimes justifiably but on other occasions quite unfairly) that surgeons developed their large and lucrative private practices at the expense of their NHS work; there are only twenty-four hours in a day after all. Conversely, there were some colleagues who worked extremely long hours with no private practice at all, who contributed all their working days to the state and therefore had a much lower annual net income.

By Merit Raised[12]

It will come as little or no surprise to the more discerning reader that the Stasi are demanding a say in who gets the bacon. This effectively means, of course, that the toadies and lickspittles get the money (completely irrespective of what they contribute, just so long as they are good boys/girls and don't blow the whistle or upset the boat).

It is very similar really to the prize system at some schools: one of your authors was always very surprised that the deportment prize at his goddaughter's school never went to one of the many African girl pupils who used to board there (often the daughters of diplomats). As he sat at school prize days watching some gawky Devon maid shuffle up to the platform to collect the annual Deportment Prize, his thoughts flew to the beautifully elegant women he had seen in Nubia carrying large earthenware pots on their heads faultlessly. His mind then flashed to those magnificent Arab race horses walking around the paddock before a race. Then he remembered for a moment with sad nostalgia how he himself was once able to balance a

---

[12]'Satan exalted sat, by merit rais'd/To that bad eminence.' John Milton, *Paradise Lost*, ll, 5.

full pint tankard on his head and bob up and down without spilling a drop whilst others in the pub would sing 'Have you seen the muffin man, who lives down Drury Lane'. These are the harlequin thoughts that flit through one's mind during those seemingly endless, unspeakably boring school prize days.

When he got home and asked his goddaughter why Maisie Woollacott[13] had won the Deportment Prize rather than Numakau, the Ethiopian ambassador's daughter, Katie laughed and told him that the prize was nothing to do with deportment, bearing and carriage of the body; it was always given to some sycophantic little teacher's pet. Maisie was evidently the biggest creep in the school, and Katie's chum Numakau would never have lived it down if she had won it!

If we shift our thoughts back to the so-called merit awards, your authors have a very good friend who has been working as a busy consultant surgeon for twenty years at a District General Hospital. He had worked there for eighteen years as the only ENT consultant at that hospital. This meant that he had been consultant-on-call every working night for eighteen years. He was not first-on-call all this time, because the hospital provided an associate specialist (a sub-consultant grade) to help out by being first-on-call on alternate nights. So here we have the extraordinary situation of a consultant being technically on-call every night of his working life for almost eighteen years and being first-on-call (i.e. the first doctor telephoned for all ENT emergencies) for alternate nights. During these years he had worked uncomplainingly doing more outpatient clinics and seeing more patients than any other firm in the hospital (and also

---

[13]The name has been changed here to protect the girl, who in truth cannot bear any of the blame for the travesty.

doing more than his fair share of operating). You would certainly be forgiven for thinking that all this work constituted 'bearing the heat and toil of the day' or working above and beyond the call of duty, but nonetheless after eighteen years he had not received any form of award at all. The more perspicacious reader may by now have guessed that the authors' friend has also had a long and distinguished record of outspoken opposition to the Stasi (including two rather acrimonious outbursts on local television and a whole scrapbook full of press releases of aspersions against 'unqualified' hospital administrators. Could his failure to merit an award perhaps be because he had not made any academic contributions? Certainly this was not the case; it could even be argued that he was the most academic consultant on the hospital staff, having taken a doctorate (MD) and an MPhil (master of philosophy) degree. He had also written four books and had a fairly impressive list of journal publications. He had lectured on ENT throughout the United Kingdom and abroad and is fairly well known in his specialty. He has been a member of national committees, and was fed up of sitting on regional and district committees and being chairman of two of the local hospitals' committees.

After nineteen years, he had still not received any sort of merit award. In fact, he was the only consultant of his degree of seniority in his hospital not to have one. What made matters worse was that two of his colleagues who had done a job-share (that means share one consultant job between the two of them) had each got one, but they were 'nice guys.' When Marcellus said, 'Something is rotten in the state of Denmark'[14] he was not referring to the Danish health system.

---

[14]*Hamlet.* Act 1, scene 4, line 90.

Just like the Deportment Prize at the school of your author's daughter has nothing to do with bearing and carriage, merit awards had little relationship to value and hard work. In fact they have changed their name in the last few years to Discretionary Awards. This is uncharacteristically honest, but at least it points out that they have nothing to do with merit. If you want one of these awards, you clearly need to toe the line and keep your mouth tightly shut. But if you choose to do this, the financial reward for sycophancy[15] is high. Many have not considered it derogatory to their dignity to exchange their self respect for a brown nose and the consideration of quite a few thousand pounds per annum (or should it be anum?).

If one is not only willing to lose one's self respect but also the respect of all one's colleagues, there are even greater financial carrots to be gleaned in the guise of the post of Medical Director. The idea of increasing the involvement of doctors in management is of course derisory to those older consultants who have been totally involved in running their own departments since they took up the post. There have been brief ups and downs in recent years in which meddlesome accountants have tried to stick their oar where it is not wanted and succeeded in ruining morale and effectively removing almost all the goodwill of the hospital staff, but the day-to-day running of clinical departments has always been effectively carried out by the clinicians. Arguably, in order to cover up the administrative incompetence and clinical impotence of the otherwise powerful accountants, the directorate system has been devised. Setting up the post of Medical Director (and

---

[15] An interesting word derived from the Greek for 'fig-blabbers' (suko-phanters). The men of Athens passed a law against exportation of figs. Of course this trade went on despite the dead-letter law, and those who blabbed to the government (for their own private ends) were known as sycophants. It later came to be a general term for a toady. In Dante's *Divine Comedy*, the deepest pit in hell was reserved for sycophants.

also subordinate Clinical Directorates) is a brilliant political ploy and provides ready scapegoats for the Stasi's mistakes. It works something like this: the chief executive appoints a highly-paid puppet 'yes man' (he has to be a consensus director – a political animal unlikely to be outspoken and very unlikely to upset any of the Stasi); he is not elected by his peers, but chosen by the Stasi. When in post this toady will, for lucre vile, take the side of management and oppose his colleagues (and as a figure his peers will be marginally less likely to hate). The price of betrayal is now much more than the traditional thirty pieces of silver.

The whole idea of appointing these Quislings[16] is far too clever for a Stasi to have conceived (as we have seen, they are invariably dullards) it must have been created by a politician. It is, of course, based on the Machiavellian[17] principle of 'Divide and Govern'[18]. The authors consider that it reflects very badly on their profession that there will always be a collaborator willing to put the love of money before duty to his patients, and sell his Hippocratic principles for a financial award. Sadly the profession continues to prostitute itself. Never mind your patients; forget about your colleagues; be an obedient party member, toe the political line and you will receive a very substantial monetary reward. A medical director is

---

[16]Vidkun Quisling, (1887–1945) was a Norwegian army officer and fascist politician, who became Minister President of Norway during the German occupation from February 1942 to the end of World War II, while the elected social democratic cabinet of Johan Nygaardsvold was exiled in London. After the war he was tried for high treason and subsequently executed by firing squad. His surname has become an eponym for 'traitor.' especially a collaborationist.

[17]Niccolò Machiavelli (1496–1527) Florentine statesman and political philosopher.

[18]Matthew, too had said, 'Every city or house divided against itself shall not stand.' (Matthew, xii; 25)

supposed 'to represent his colleagues' but clearly this can never be the case because the type of consultant who is interested in taking on this office is clearly not representative of his colleagues, otherwise he would not apply!

Finally it has been suggested that granting financial awards (which they will continue to receive until retirement and will be pensionable) to doctors undertaking management duties represents paying them three times![xii] Firstly because it has always been an implicit and essential part of every consultant's job that he will be undertaking a certain amount of management duties anyway; secondly because in the new set-up, the consultant will be dropping clinical sessions (which still need to be done) and being given extra remuneration for Stasi duties; and thirdly by the 'gentleman's agreement' he will get a discretionary award in due course.

At the end of the day of course it boils down to what a consultant wants from life. Some are happy working at a district hospital, fishing, golfing or growing sweet peas; others choose to scale the heights of academia or plumb the depths of politics.

Handrails or Handcuffs?

It is generally held that a better educated and trained medical workforce will provide a better standard of health care. It is unfortunate then that the very people who urge us to go on study leave, attend courses, etc, often have control of the purse strings and have to withhold permission or funding (which usually amounts to the same thing) to do this[19]. As the reader will have

---

[19]Comparison can be made with policemen who so cherish their status as keepers of the peace and protectors of the public that they have occasionally been known to beat to death those citizens or groups who question that status. Foreign policemen, that is.

probably come to realise by now, this rarely happens. Money that is specially allocated for training is often 'raided' to balance the books elsewhere. The authors have no proof that it has ever been used to send 'executives' on paint-balling or other forms of 'bonding' exercises, but this does not mean to say that it hasn't! Professor Sir Miles Irving of the University of Manchester, who has sat on many Government Committees on this subject, considers that the supervision and ultimate control of the process should remain fairly and squarely in the hands of the medical profession.[xiii]

The ultra-cynical, the ultimate example of whom must surely be F.M. Cornford, may agree with his aphorism that 'Plainly, the more rules you can invent, the less need there will be to waste time over fruitless puzzling over right and wrong.'[xiv] It has been pointed out, however, (and those with experience of the former Eastern European government bureaucracies will confirm this) that blind obedience to 'rules' leads to the situation where the consequence is that half the things are done twice, the other half not done at all. Rules have to be interpreted and the performance of jobs put into some of order (what people like to call 'prioritised').

Of course, rules can be very useful for those who seek refuge behind them. Blind to their inner reason, they can then justify their actions by 'I was only following orders.'[20] Are we, as doctors, immune to this form of mass hysteria? Remember, World War II only too tragically showed how it can overtake whole nations. People can, under special circumstances, actually take part in the most bizarre acts even in these enlightened times – Morris

---

[20]At SS Obersturmbannfuhrer Adolf Eichmann's (illegal) trial in 1962, he explicitly declared that he had abdicated his conscience in order to follow the Führerprinzip: *'Befehlt ist Befehlt'* ('Orders are orders!'). He was later executed.

dancing springs immediately to mind. The example of this 'more than my job's worth' mentality which most often comes to mind for doctors is the rule 'retrospective claims will not be allowed.' This is even when they have lost your original request, of which you have proof of submission, a copy and a receipt. There are some things in this world which we will probably never fully understand no matter how much continuing medical education we undertake.

CHAPTER 6

PEOPLE ARE MORE IMPORTANT THAN PLACES

The Modern Architecture Hospital

Your authors have been privileged to work in Victorian buildings in the North of England that were built with some sort of community pride (even if they did start out life as workhouses). They had proportion, presence, showed architectural good manners (even though they stood separate from the rows of houses surrounding) and, in contrast to most modern buildings *you could find the front door*. For those doubting Thomases, just go to a modern theatre, library, courthouse or whatever and see where the front door is meant to be. Far from being at the focus of the building it is invariably hidden. When finally located, it will be seen to consist of four or more pieces of glass masquerading as doors. One less than the total (for mathematicians this might be represented as $n - 1$) will have grubby pieces of paper with the words 'Use Other Door' scribbled on. We have yet to find 'Use Other Door's', but it cannot be long in coming.[1]

---

[1]Your authors do not want to appear as curmudgeons (perish the thought!) but while we are on this rant, has the reader never considered that the correct instructions for those ghastly hand heaters (dryers?) to be found in public conveniences should be 'shake hands dry, agitate under the stream of hot air, then dry off by wiping on the arse of your trousers'?

Why don't these designers live and work in their creations? Instead, they seem to refurbish warehouses, watermills and such like. Have they no faith in their work? We have an answer for them. Stop what you are doing, experience what trouble you wreak and do the decent thing. Loaded revolvers should be provided in strategic places.

An aphorism used in the advertising world (the word 'world' being a useful compromise between trade and profession!) is that one is 'not selling the sausage, but the sizzle'. Corporate identity is all-important: logos abound whilst wards are neglected. 'No Smoking' signs are also seen in profusion – this might not necessarily be a bad thing, and might well be a result of the firm making all the other signs, headed writing paper, etc, being given a free hand to increase its profits. Should that be the case, then where are all the *No Spitting* signs beloved of the authors' childhood? Or why not take a page out of the Frenchman's book? Outpatient Department walls might become decorated with '*Défense d'uriner*'! We surely do not want customers (patients) to urinate over everything (unless perhaps it is a urology clinic). It can only be a question of time before some enterprising person, supported by legal aid, challenges his right not to be prevented from doing this, as it is not specifically prohibited.

Your authors do not want to descend into a slough of despond, but consider William Morris's Address to the Anti Scrape Society, 1889[2]:

---

[2]'The Anti Scrape Brigade' was more properly called the Society for the Protection of Ancient Buildings. Morris's staunch ally in leading this campaign was the famous Gothic Revivalist, John Ruskin. By the nineteenth century, church walls had been rendered by many successive coats of plastering and 'the Victorian 'restorers' had discovered that by hacking off this 'dishonest' plaster, all sorts of architectural treasures, bricked up like nuns were once again brought to light. More often than not however, nothing was found and disastrous results came from what Morris called 'skinning a church alive'. (For a fuller account, see J. Riddington Young, 2000)

Just consider what England was in the fourteenth century. The population ... At about four millions. Think then of the amount of beautiful and dignified buildings which those four millions built .... Not only those churches and houses which we see, but also those which have been destroyed .... Those buildings .... contained much art: pictures, metal-work, carvings, tapestry and the like, altogether forming a prodigious mass of art, produced by a scanty population. Try to imagine that.

What people seem not to realize now is that work is done better and more efficiently if the workers are in pleasant surroundings – if their hospital feels a part of the community, fits well into the town, if the writing paper bears the hospital crest (if the hospital still has a crest), if there is a hospital tie, etc.

What is it about the modern office worker (and remember that although we might dress up the term as 'consulting rooms', to all intents and purposes that is where we spend a great deal of our time) that makes him put up with such awful surroundings? Surely there is some room for a little decoration? By that, your authors do not mean those stupid little executive toys whereby balls suspended from a beam are caused to bang into one another, thus demonstrating that although superhuman work is done here by people with intellects of extra-terrestrial proportions, the humble laws of the universe such as gravity, etc, are still obeyed. Or perhaps the jaded executive is simply bored with the sound of his own thought processes. He would probably 'customise' his car by buying the factory-fitted option of alloy wheels so that his car can look the same as everybody else's who has n thousands of pounds (where n is a large number) to waste. Yet would he pay a real artist to create something unique for him, and to his taste – assuming such an artist could be found.

The freedom to express oneself is becoming more and more curtailed through the nature of the materials with which things are made and the method by which we pay for objects. Nobody dare alter the plastic fascia of a car (it would be difficult to do anyway) for fear of harming the resale value. How many people actually use the ashtray? – yet very few have the skill or means (despite years of woodwork classes, ha ha) at school. Woodwork? – not one in a hundred could actually wield a tenon saw successfully and 'customise' a fitted kitchen. You take what you can get, and are grateful. Of course the modern executive (and that is what the Stasi consider themselves to be) has a profound need to demonstrate individualism. The trouble is that he can only feel at ease doing this by wearing a bright yellow patterned tie or Donald Duck socks. He thus establishes himself as a free-thinking, modern, approachable 'one of the guys' – like all those others who can spare some ghastly chain shop the right amount of money to be similarly kitted-out. One of your authors had the good sense and taste to commission a beautiful Art Nouveau desk plaque for his name plate instead of the hideous plastic job issued after the correct number of requisition forms, authorities and dockets had been completed. It is a beautiful piece, which gave work to the artist, satisfaction to the person who bought it as a present and joy to its owner. It was recently admired by one of the clones who lives his life out of a mail-order catalogue; he said he would make a mental note to acquire something similar. Your author restrained himself from asking: 'A mental note? – on what?'

The Car Park Question

At the 1999 BMA Conference the incredible fact came to light that most junior doctors are charged for parking their motor cars at the hospital where they work. Since they are now often expected to work at more than one hospital, and the Trusts expect them to have a car, they claimed it was unfair that they should have to pay at all and asked for reserved parking places.[i]

Things have got a lot worse since then. The mercenary nature of the Stasi will by now have been made apparent and when it was realized that making charges for car-parking presented a chance for amassing wealth beyond even their own dreams of avarice[3], this opportunity was rapidly seized upon.

The fact that it is clearly immoral (Macmillan Cancer Relief said it was 'morally wrong' to raise revenue by forcing patients to pay for parking) and unethical to change parking fees to the sick or to visitors cuts no ice. Believe it or not, some hospitals make £1.5million a year by extorting money from the ill and their relatives for the wonderful privilege of parking in an NHS car park.[ii]

Pity Janine, the poor wife of the victim in the London Terrorist bomb attack in July 2006. Her husband[4] was blown up and lost a leg and was admitted to the Royal Free Hospital. Somewhat distraught after a harrowing 400-mile drive from Yorkshire to come and visit her loved one, she was made to waste over half an hour driving round looking for a parking space. When she eventually found somewhere to leave her car so that she could

---

[3]Dr Samuel Johnson the famous lexicographer was a very special friend of Mrs. Thrale, wife of the owner of Thrales' Brewery. He was involved with its sale and is reported to have said to some prospective buyers: 'Gentlemen, we are not here to sell a parcel of vats and boilers, but the potential of becoming rich beyond the dreams of avarice.' Time was certainly to prove him right; Thrales eventually became Courage Breweries.

[4]Your authors as doctors certainly refuse to use the word 'partner' when 'spouse', 'husband', 'wife', 'lover', 'boyfriend' etc is actually meant. Doctors and lawyers to whom the word has a long established and precise meaning (and indeed most intelligent educated persons) shun such incorrect usage.

eventually see her husband, it cost her in excess of £3 an hour for one of its limited number of parking spaces – and she wasn't allowed to stay for more than a few hours at time. Then during his stay, Janine, who kept a round-the-clock vigil at her husband's bed for the first few days, found herself regularly having to leave his side to deal with the car.

Car parking charges alone amounted to around £36 a day – but that was nothing compared with the stress generated by having frantically to search for a new space every few hours. Janine regularly had to leave the hospital car park, and search for a meter in a side street as close to the hospital as possible.[iii]

The girls on the front desk at the hospital where one of your authors worked tell heart-breaking stories of old ladies in tears because they have not got the money or the right change for the meters so that they can visit their sick and ailing husbands.

Perhaps more surprising, though arguably not quite as immoral (at the risk, again, of appearing pedantic, it is unethical rather than immoral), the girls on the desk are themselves expected to pay to park their own cars at the hospital where they work. The charge per person per car is £87.50 per annum. A few years ago, when your author was appointed as a consultant, he was allocated a designated space marked 'Consultant ENT'. He continued to use this space for over twenty years, but last year when he returned to his car at 8 o'clock in the evening after a busy afternoon in the operating theatre, he found that it had been wheel-clamped! He drives a geriatric Jaguar (not quite in the same league as the late lamented Inspector Morse) and when he rang up the Director of Facilities, he was actually informed that they had been trying to immobilise his car (presumably whilst he had been working for the good of his patients in the hospital) for over a year! 'We tried the other clamps and even tried chaining your wheels, but it just didn't work; they just wouldn't fit that old thing of yours!' They had eventually bought a special clamp that would fit a sixteen-year-old Jag. They actually sounded very pleased with themselves. When it was tactfully pointed out that he was on call, the Director of Facilities said that he could not possibly give the porters authority to remove the clamp and his best advice was to pay the unclamping fee of £20 and claim it back on his 'On-Call' claim form!

The following morning, JRY rang the General Manager of the Surgical and Anaesthetics Directorate (a pleasant middle aged woman who used to work in an Accountants' Office in Bideford) to claim back his money for attending the hospital whilst he was 'On-Call' for Surgical Emergencies. 'I am sorry' she said, 'You have to pay to park even if you are called in by the hospital to see an emergency!' When JRY told her that he had recorded this statement, she became most indignant, and told him that he had no right to do so. Let us hope she can now see it for herself. Your author did not actually record his reply to her but they were somewhere along the lines of, 'I would rather crawl to work on my hands and knees over broken glass than pay to park where I work.' Since that time, he has parked a distance from work and walks to his office (on his feet)!

Even more outrageous is the tale of a young Casualty Officer at another hospital in the West Country, who arrived at work but could not find anywhere to park. She spent over half an hour driving round until she was contacted by an irate sister of Casualty Theatre on her cell phone to tell her that her first patient was ready and waiting for his anaesthetic. Rather than incur the wrath of Sister and hold the theatre list up, she really stuck her neck out and parked her car in the reserved Stasi's car park. Mere doctors are clearly not important enough to have a reserved spot.

During the course of the first surgical operation, the outraged Stasi whose space had been used had the temerity to stick his head around the door of the Operating Theatre and demand that the offending car be removed as soon as possible or it would be wheel-clamped! The reader will be delighted to learn that she told him in the politest terms she could muster that her first priority would be to her patients and that she would finish her operating list before moving her car. Her car was not clamped.

We are waiting for the day when some highly-paid management guru (or consultant) will come to the conclusion that having such privileged parking spaces right outside their place of work will save each doctor fifteen minutes per day which would otherwise have been wasted looking for a place and which can now be used in the care of patients. We expect to have to wait a long time.

The Noise Question

Music and pleasurable sounds have always figured large in human life and happiness, and unpleasant noise such as alarm clocks and air raid sirens can produce a contrasting irritation. This is especially so when one is lying peacefully asleep, or ill in bed. This was well known in the past when straw would be strewn over the cobbles to muffle the noise of passing horses and carts. In more recent memory, your authors (as children) remember a road sign at the approach to every British hospital: it was supposed to be a symbol of a flaming torch[5] but looked more to us like a Mr Whippy ice cream cornet. Somewhat later, signs in the immediate hospital vicinity stated 'Quiet Please – Hospital'. This may seem to the inpatient of today a rather hollow joke and

---

[5] It was a bit like that tacky Tory Party logo around the late 1990s.

modern hospitals may be better likened to the hustle and bustle of a shopping centre[6] than the quiet restful settings exemplified in nursing home advertisements. In particular, the problem found in many hospitals is that the gardens have now been turned over to car parks. The low gentle rumble of background traffic noise may well be bearable to the sedated sick and staff but a more irritating sound which constantly assails the ears nowadays is that of the car alarms which are continually being set off.

The background noise in an average general ward varies between 45 and 70 dB[iv] – this compares favourably with that found in everyday life – for example 65–85 in a restaurant or hairdressing salon but is not so good as a park (40–50dB) or library (35dB).[v] On the other hand (in former times) when the consultant was doing his ward round levels have been found to drop to that of a church (30dB) – which is in fact the recommended level for wards during the night.[vi] In contrast the alarm clock by the side of the bed produces a sound at ear level of anything from 85–100dB.

All of your authors wear (proper) leather shoes and one of them was told by his mother that he should have little metal inserts put in the back of his heels to prolong the life of the shoes. He has to confess that he still follows mater's advice but admits that this does indeed cause a characteristic clicking sound when he enters the ward, a fact that for many years has been very useful to the nursing staff as a sort of early warning system. About twenty years ago, he was somewhat surprised to see a circular from the Stasi suggesting that in order to reduce

---

[6]Of course, many hospitals do now have more in common with commercial retail centres than places where the sick may be treated owing to the possibilities of generating income from rent charged to shops.

noise levels on the wards, quieter shoes are worn by all staff. He replied to this notice by circulating his own suggestions (and from no less than an ear specialist) that the best way to reduce noise levels would be deep shag-pile carpets on all the ward floors and that special *anechoic* tiling on the walls would also help. Because these tiles would be so expensive, compressed cardboard egg-cartons would be a good substitute. To defray expenses then, perhaps the staff could all bring in their used egg boxes which could be deposited at certain designated collection points in the hospital for attachment later to the ward walls. The Chief Executive wrote to tell him that she thought his circular was 'not helpful'.

The Dining Room

It is the accepted wisdom now that not only should all workers eat together, but that hospital dining rooms should also be open to relatives, and, by extension, any member of the public who happens to drop by. This is all very well and good, but the authors wonder what would happen should they call in at their local police station, fire station or law courts and try to exercise the same privilege.

Of course, things have not always been bad – or perhaps people used to be more easily satisfied. Witness the conversation overheard by a friend in a Royal Air Force Medical Officers' Mess:

> I hear old Carruthers is applying for permission to get married.
>   Why, doesn't he like living in the Mess?

This may be taking the idea of the institution as 'family' a little too far, but was it really so bad for medical colleagues to meet over lunch? Nowadays one barely knows one's fellow consultants and a referral of a case is quite impersonal. The medical chat that used to go on is now impossible in the common eating areas which include the general public, and most doctors seem now to live off sandwiches eaten at their desk. When the Doctors' Dining Rooms were first closed (on the grounds that they were élitist), arguments were put forward that doctors would now have no place to go to discuss patients' problems in a confidential and secure environment. The hospital was the 'home' of the housemen for a large part of their week and now they no longer had their own dining room but had to queue up with the public in a cafeteria. This cut no ice. As usual, the plan was to save money despite any upset to the real workers in the hospital.

Those who know no different will not miss anything. This is just like so much of hospital life. It is clear that one cannot aspire to something one knows nothing about. The old Consultants' Dining Room, which was a bit like a Gentleman's Club[7] (often boasting a very fine wine cellar), was perhaps inevitably doomed as an anachronism. What criticism could possibly be levelled at the 'paternal' consultant, however who ran 'his' department with personal pride, took an interest in 'his' junior medical colleagues, nurses and medical students alike, raised money for 'his' ward. The hospital was rather like an extended family. He is about as dead as a dodo. He has been killed by the new commercial ethos.

Newcomers to the profession will have not experienced him or anyone like him and so will be content to be merely commuters, living at home and doing the work required (the sessions they are contracted for) and then returning home again. They would never dream of mixing their social life with their 'work' (NB in the past,

---

[7]Not that it ever excluded lady doctors, but their spouses might have found difficulty in gaining admission.

it would have been their profession). They do not even want to be involved in medical educational meetings if they are not held during working hours. After all they can be kept up to date with the Internet! The modern medics will no longer be the backbone of the hospital which used to be a thriving community of wards, clinics, residences, dining rooms and the social club.

The Stasi will have won.

Patient Advocacy

God defend me from my friends; from my enemies
I can defend myself.

Fifteenth century proverb

That their heart is in the right place cannot be denied, but it can be said that the blind pursuit of the perfect is the enemy of achieving the good and adequate. In this, the case of children in hospital might be considered. In a (superficially very laudable) attempt to improve the conditions of children in hospital, some pressure groups have made it very difficult for them to be treated at all. This is especially the case in small or district hospitals where for the lack of an 'age-appropriate toy' or some other failing of the many regulations now in force, all paediatric services are transferred miles away. It can be a difficult choice and one which the authors have much sympathy for. What we cannot understand is how the medical profession – and often the patients themselves – have very little say in the choices to be made. 'Suffer the little children' indeed.

Despite this, it must not be thought that the monopoly of patient advocacy lies with the lay public. Perhaps we should distinguish between patient advocacy and political or financial expediency.

Doctors have long been at the forefront of speaking up for more resources to be allocated to the sick and needy. Some might have written this as 'allocated to healthcare'. The social reformer and artist Käthe Kollwitz (1867–1945), who was the wife of a doctor, wrote and drew in the most eloquent terms the problems facing the poor in Germany before, during and after World War I. One of her most moving pictures concerns a mother bringing her infant (who clearly is suffering from tuberculosis) to the doctor. It is entitled 'At the Doctor's' and is a part of a pamphlet 'Against Exploitation'. Unfortunately, the copyright fee is excessive (which, considering the title, is somewhat ironic!) and so, although it was reproduced in a thesis[8], it cannot be shown here. However, the text follows:

> Doctor: The sick boy is greatly undernourished. He needs daily milk, eggs, meat and fat.
> Mother: Doctor, I do not have the money. I am not even able to buy all the food available on coupons.
> Doctor: This way, usury and profiteering make our youth perish.
>
> *
>
> Are you able to watch this without doing anything against it? Everyone should help in battling this, the worst enemy of the people. Denounce all profiteering to the police or courts. All civil lawyers and police authorities accept notifications. National Police Office at the State Commission for Nutrition

Perhaps we should not get too hot under the collar about social deprivation – unless we are the sort of person who is happy

---

[8]Bennett J D C. *Doctors, Patients, and Power*. University of Wales MA, 1996.

shouldering the world's burdens. Thank goodness there are such people (Kollwitz's husband was a doctor and she obviously had much contact with the poor). Yet, as George Bernard Shaw points out: 'Doctoring is not the art of keeping people in health (no doctor seems able to advise you what to eat any better than his grandmother or the nearest quack): it is the art of curing illnesses.'

An Old Poacher Makes the Best Keeper[9]

One chairman of the Patients' Association proved the old adage about the converted poacher; he had previously been the Chief Executive of the Brighton Health Care Trust. The tenure of Dr John Spiers[10] was distinguished by two really well-conceived and highly intelligent deeds (which our readers will have by now come to expect from a Stasi!). One very good idea was to test the attitude of the Trust to disabled people. He clearly thought it would be a very meaningful and useful exercise and would also put the under-worked doctors and nurses of the Brighton Casualty Department on their mettle. His carefully conceived plan involved presenting himself to the casualty department and pretending to be completely paralysed from the waist down. Our readers will not be too surprised to learn that the Trust Chairman was not recognised by any of the staff.

But it would appear that he was rumbled!

Had he done his homework properly, he would have found out that even a very junior doctor should be able to distinguish a

---

[9]Fourteenth-century proverb.

[10]Perhaps we should clarify the 'doctor' business: John Spiers received a D.Mus. (hon.) from Sussex University (it is generally considered non-U to use the title 'doctor' when honorary – particularly when working in a hospital where there are a lot of physicians about). Your authors will refrain from any interpretation of his motives in this respect.

malingerer from a hysteric[11] (and certainly both of these from somebody suffering an actual true paralysis). Evidently nobody was very impressed by his play acting and he was left on a trolley to meditate for a short while (which was probably part of his treatment). Anyway, he soon became cold and bored, and so started to berate a hospital porter for not wearing his name badge, which he told him was in contravention of the Patients' Charter. The porter too had clearly not recognised the elevated personage who was reprimanding him and told him to f**k off![12] This perhaps underlines the importance in leadership of being known to your men.

Apparently Dr Spiers did not enjoy his visit. He was evidently appalled by the filthy state of the walls and lights; he was horrified to find that he had no pillow on his trolley, and had to be moved to another cubicle because the first one let the rain in. He experienced despair when he was told there may be a five-hour wait for a doctor. His teeth chattered with cold and he felt ashamed of the lack of privacy and dignity he was made to endure in the hospital of which *he* was CEO. Through all that suffering, however, there came enlightenment. Dr Spiers realised he had discovered 'the invisible hospital' that management never sees![13]

---

[11]For the benefit of any Stasi persevering, a malingerer is a plain old-fashioned lead-swinger, but a hysteric is mentally ill rather than physically ill, and believes himself to have something (usually very serious) wrong with himself.

[12]*Sunday Times*, 24 April 1994 pp 4–8.

[13]He has written an amazingly readable book called *The Invisible Hospital and the Secret Garden*; in this he defines the Secret Garden as 'the private world of professionals, which is unknown, untouched and unaccountable to ordinary people' (Spiers. *The Invisible Hospital and the Secret Garden – An Insider's Commentary on the NHS Reforms*. Radcliffe Medical Press, Oxford: 1995. p xxii). Our favourite quotation from this is, 'Patient involvement is vital if health care is to be a genuine therapeutic relationship.' We have not made this up – it really says it! (on page 159).

Your authors believe that he is a well-meaning man who went through with this pantomime with the best intentions. They also think it is a great pity that it took this elaborate charade for him to realise what an underfunded shambles the casualty department had become. Had he asked the casualty consultant, or even a casualty house officer, sister or nurse (or for that matter, the porter without the name badge) working there, they would have all been able to tell him.

Spiers' response to his day in casualty is an eloquent example of how the mind of a Stasi works. After his enlightenment, he tried (bless him!) to help. Having realised that the casualty department was understaffed, underfunded, letting rain and water into the cubicles, he set out to help put things right. He did not, however, inject any cash into casualty by getting extra hands to the pumps and employing a few more workers (doctors and nurses) so that a patient might see a doctor without having to wait for five hours or that more time could be spent talking to patients (even mentally sick ones who have pretended to have lost the use of their legs!). No! He did not do anything as obvious as that. What he did do was truly inspired.

He set up a Patients' Access Group to involve patients in policy making, and he set up the first ever, full-time *Patients' Advocate*, employed exclusively to take up casualty patients' complaints on their behalf.

This way of thinking speaks volumes about the upside-down thought processes of the Stasi and the philosophy that he shows here is absolutely typical of the ethos and values of senior hospital management. Anyone other than a Stasi would surely understand that an injured patient arriving at a casualty department (particularly one who is not pretending, but is genuinely terrified and in fear of his life) is not really concerned about a Patients'

Advocate or whether the porter is wearing a name badge.[14] It is our honest belief that sick people would be better pleased with more doctors and nurses on the ground to give rapid and effective treatment, comfort and reassurance.

Perhaps one of the reasons why he didn't want to employ any more doctors is because he has a deep seated dislike (or even paranoid envy?) of hospital doctors. Paradoxically, he considers that consultants are 'arrogant' and 'rude' and 'unable to relate to' and 'communicate clearly' with 'ordinary people'.[vii] This hurtful generalisation is particularly ironic coming from a Chief Executive, since poor communication skills and insufferable arrogance had always appeared to us to be two of the distinguishing hallmarks of the Stasi.

In 1994, however, Dr Spiers really overstepped the mark with verbal abuse of his betters, when perhaps his most famous quotation appeared in the *BMA News Review* under the heading THE MAN DOCTORS LOVE TO HATE[viii]. He started his interview saying that doctors 'had powers but no accountability'. This didn't really upset anyone (perhaps because it is no longer true); then he said doctors 'have lived in a secret garden. It's my view that softly softly has not caught the monkey'. This too certainly did not upset anybody, perhaps because nobody knew what on earth he was talking about. Spiers antagonised the nation's doctors by actually going on to say that he 'would not choose to travel in a railway carriage' with consultants from the Brighton Hospital. Now our readers might think those doctors at the hospital in Brighton were being over sensitive, but Spiers

---

[14]In 1905, the newly built Casualty Department of the Royal Hospital, West Street, Sheffield, did not waste money on Patients' Advocates. They set up a huge painted notice on the wall of the casualty waiting room. It said: "I moaned because I had no shoes, until one day I met a man who had no feet – Chinese proverb."

statement of tact, diplomacy and obvious refined discrimination[15] was not well received by some of them, who, though they might well have shared the sentiment[16] considered that it was somewhat disrespectful and inappropriate for national publication. A vote of no confidence was proposed at the Medical Executive Meeting, and would have been unanimous, but the Medical Director declined to support the motion (see also the previous chapter – Quislings). He then left as Chairman of the Trust and became Chairman of the Patients' Association. He has since left them too.

Advertising

In the past, the worth of a doctor was based not so much on reputation as self-proclamation (in stark contrast to nowadays, of course). It is difficult to split eighteenth-century medical practitioners into professionals and traders solely on the basis of their performance.[ix] In the free-for-all, regular practitioners

---

[15]Which your authors try to show at all times.

[16]Before the days of commercial television and advertising breaks between programmes (US: 'messages'), the BBC used a number of short films that were shown during these intermissions. They were usually entitled 'Interlude'. Perhaps the best known was a tank full of angel fish just swimming around. Others included a potter at work at his wheel making a vase, a kitten playing with a ball of wool and there was a rather boring one of a windmill. Your authors' favourite, however, was called 'London to Brighton in two minutes' and was a film taken from a camera on the front of the train from London to Brighton and then speeded up to last for two minutes precisely and accompanied by Rimsky-Korsakov's 'Flight of the Bumble Bee'. One of your authors was cruelly duped by his brother, abetted by his father, (at the time he was about eight years of age) that this was the actual duration of the journey and the express was a very fast train. He suffered from this delusion for many years, before his father told him the truth. The real journey time is even now (i.e. forty years on) about fifty minutes. Thus spending the time in the company of someone from the shallow end of the gene pool (e.g. a Stasi) could prove to be a harrowing experience.

had to compete with quack itinerants, nostrum-vendors, and empirics.[x] Often the only way to convince the rest of the world of your worth was to enlist the help of clever writers and friends to spread the word.

By contrast, in the Victorian era the rise of professionalism via bureaucratic or state control gradually replaced market mechanisms,[xi] and the professionalisation of medicine served to strengthen control and to rescue the profession from the undignified bogland of the medical market.[xii] It is traditionally considered that State Regulations were introduced to reform the boundaries of the medical profession – examples would be the Apothecaries Act of 1815 and the Medical Act of 1858.[xiii] The profession itself developed a strong moral code:

> That it is undesirable that any Fellow or member of the College should be officially connected with any Company having for its object the treatment of disease for profit.
>
> Resolution of the Royal College of Physicians of London,
> 25 Oct 1888

However, whilst consultants could dictate this sort of behaviour, they themselves built up large lucrative practices on the basis of their 'voluntary' work in the teaching hospitals. It seems that there was considerable intra-professional struggle whereby non-élite doctors tried to find methods of breaking the monopoly of the élite – often by seeking other methods of financial gain.[xiv] This included endorsing advertisements and joining laymen's medical businesses. As competition created a downward pressure on medical incomes,[xv] it was not unknown for suicide to occur... Clearly such people have forgotten Samuel Johnson's dictum in his *Life of Sir Thomas Browne*:

The physician's part lies hid in domestic privacy, and silent duties and silent excellencies are soon forgotten.

He also held that 'no man but a blockhead ever wrote except for money'[xvi] – it should be remembered that he was arrested for debt the very year that his great dictionary had, after many years of labour, been published.

The Time and Motion Men

We can easily count the number of operations performed correctly or even the number of correct operations performed. With a little imagination it may even be possible to count the number of correct operations performed correctly on the correct patients from the correct waiting list.

But surgical performance, like love, is often in the eye of the beholder. In the good old days (whenever that may have been), a surgeon regarded his performance as not quite as good as it might have been, were it not for all those dreadful committees he had to attend (and which he probably volunteered for) and also because of the management which had denied him proper facilities. His performance, however, would have been far better than that of his colleagues. Of these colleagues, the older ones would now be slowing down and were really almost past it; and the younger ones would still be wet behind the ears. Yes, self-confidence has always been the hallmark of a surgeon. That and a profound sense of one's position in the scheme of things. One is reminded of the conjugation of the reflexive verb 'to be firm':

I am firm,
You are stubborn,
He is pig-headed.

Whilst operating, surgeons can find themselves using its sibling:

I am speedy yet cautious,
You are cavalier,
He is a cowboy.

Forty-four years perhaps represents one year's experience repeated forty-three times.[xvii] The wise, kindly physician recounting his accumulated wisdom in such a manner is probably not likely to do well in these days of self-proclaiming. How then should we judge? There are various performance indicators, but these, like so many things, need to be interpreted with care. An unpunctual man is always in a hurry; but it does not follow that hurry is the cause of unpunctuality.[xviii] Tests are administered by, in the main, non-surgical (and non-medical) people. In the manner beloved of those Latin lessons: question expecting the answer yes – *nonne*, question expecting the answer no – *num*, the answer required can be elicited by clever framing of the study and the questions asked. How quick? How many complications? There are even methods of putting a value on time, loss of amenity etc. By reducing everything to one common currency (i.e. currency) the money men can assess the performance of each and every surgeon. How much money in? How much money spent? That is all very well if all surgeons did one or two well-defined procedures. It might be a good way of assessing the performance of a chain of replacement tyre and exhaust shops. But what about the surgeon who does something else other than two routine operations?

Homing in on one specific procedure, it is extraordinarily difficult to prove statistically that one procedure is better than another. Sometimes, of course, events overtake one: the highly decorated Lt Col Nick Downie DSO MBE MC recounts how he was examining a man in the home guard.[xix] He found nothing seriously wrong with him, chatted about the man's vegetable garden and prescribed a benign medicine. The man thanked him, smiled, saluted, and dropped dead. This, one hopes, is the exception and we are usually in the hands of the statisticians. With their characteristic love of jargon, it would probably read something like, 'in order to obtain sufficient power, the numbers in each limb must be enormous.' Imagine the complicating factors comparing two surgeons – with different operating days, anaesthetists, juniors etc. One cannot get away from the fact that the wrong operation performed well one hundred times is still wrong. The right operation done wrongly is also wrong.

Yet people with little knowledge of medicine and even less of surgical procedures direct (or try to direct) which patients should be operated on and when. If the hospital statistics are looking unfavourable, and some Stasi might not get her (or occasionally his) bonus, then difficult procedures on very ill patients are abandoned for quick through-put easy cases.

One of the great initial benefits of the NHS was the absence of any financial incentive, or any spare operating time, for a surgeon to perform a less than necessary operation – not only to the hazard of the patient but also to the detriment of the needy – however enthusiastically sought by the patient. This is in contrast to countries where recompense is more directly related to 'output'. The 'market' and 'customer' philosophy, together with the mindless number-massaging 'waiting list initiatives' are in danger of jeopardising this.

CHAPTER 7

THE NEW LANGUAGE

If Language Is Imprecise

If language is imprecise or incorrect, then what is said is not
what is meant; and if what is said is not what is meant, then
what ought to be done remains undone.

Confucius[1]

It is a danger when writing of such matters that one might
become very pedantic and an intellectual snob. There are people
who seem to manage to lead happy productive lives who do not
know that 'didcots' are the paper residue left after holes have
been punched in paper so that it can be put into a folder. It is not
the main purpose of this book to ram enlightenment down the
throats of those who may choose to risk health and happiness on

---

[1]This aphorism appeared on the front of the *Army Staff College Guide to More Efficient
English*, given to one of your authors when attending Staff College. This surprised the
other author, who did not know that Confucius could speak English.

this long and weary road to the grave by remaining ignorant of this fact. Though, by reading the above, they have somewhat jeopardised this experiment. Nevertheless, it is clear that in today's NHS there is a new jargon being created.

We are not talking about the simple perversity of the English language, though perverse it often can be. Many of our readers are aware of the so-called 'mobile telephone'. Yet what mobility does it possess? Placed on a flat surface, it will (in the authors' experience and paranormal phenomena excepted) remain there. It is not a mobile telephone at all, but a portable one – as demonstrated all the time by those horrid people who *carry* it about. In contrast, there exist in hospitals enormous lumps of metal requiring an electric motor to propel them along even flat surfaces: these can hardly be called portable X-ray machines. *Mobile* might well fit the bill here. Anyway, as we said earlier, this is not the sort of thing we want to consider (though this example is something one of the authors has wanted to get off his chest for ages).

Let us start at the top. What is HealthCare? It is a neologism which found its way into the dictionary only at the time of printing.[2] Presumably it is meant to mean the care of 'ill people'; though it might be thought of as 'conservation' of health. We feel we know what they are getting at – but when your authors were at school and activities such as reading, writing, spelling and arithmetic were being assessed, we could not rely on this defence. The schoolmaster appended a tick (good) or cross (bad) in the margin. Nobody was ever so bold as to suggest that 'he knew what one was getting at'. If it wasn't clear, concise and correct, then it was wrong. And we were mere schoolboys (mod:

---

[2] Though with the ridiculous capital letter C in tact.

'schoolkids'). How unfortunate that someone so young, and an amateur (the worst form of insult nowadays) should be judged so rigorously, whilst the advertising megalomaniacs, spin doctors and public relations gurus get off so lightly with their *HealthCare*. They mean treatment of the sick. Note also the change in the word 'quality'. It has been contracted to stand for good or high quality. When one speaks of, for example, quality HealthCare, the implication is that it is high quality.

One of your authors was bemused to find in a series of communications from the administration of a District General Hospital, in a town not generally noted for its high ambient intelligent quotient, in the North-West of England, the repeated use of the word 'proleptic'[3]. It seemed to appear in every other memorandum, notice and the various other exhortations to greater productivity that daily fill the in-tray of the average clinician. Your author began to seriously wonder whether a new standard use of English was being attempted. He need not have worried. He received a note regarding a question posed about some treatment given to a patient by his predecessor, the gist of the notes being:

> Referred to ENT surgeons with a view to biopsy of a lymph node in the neck. FBC and ESR normal... I took a fine needle aspirate... admission for endoscopy... He is being admitted this week for panendoscopy and I will repeat the fine needle aspirate. Discharge sheet: Panendoscopy FNA swelling (L) neck – pus.

---

[3]Prolepsis: anticipation 1. A rhetorical device by which objections are anticipated and answered in advance; 2. Use of a word after a verb in anticipation of its becoming applicable through the action of the verb. (*Collins English Dictionary and Thesaurus*, Glasgow: Harper Collins, 1993 p 913.)

The Stasi had written:

Translation please. We do not understand the abbreviations used and are not exactly sure what panendoscopy relates to.

One hopes he was not one of those few Stasi (see also Quisling) who hold a medical qualification. Your author restrained himself from writing:

ENT Ear, Nose & Throat
FBC Full blood count
ESR Erythrocyte sedimentation rate
(L) Left
Panendoscopy – this is an operation; if you have five or so years to spare then you can study this (and others) at Medical School.

The medical historian, Irvine Loudon wrote eloquently in the British Medical Journal[i] how the word 'nosocomial' (as in 'nosocomial infection') is derived from an obsolete French word *nosocome* meaning hospital. This is according to the *Oxford English Dictionary* (the big one, not the concise). Dorland's *American Illustrated Medical Dictionary* (21st edition) says that it is derived from two Greek words meaning 'disease' and 'to take care of'. No problems will occur if the reader represses any urge to use *nosocomial* and instead substitutes the word 'hospital'.

Special names can be used to hide things – as is shown by the term Rapid Erection Medical Shelters (REMS). The authors think that these may be tents which cost so very much that such a simple title might set the National Audit Office worrying.

Special Clinic in Scotland

The same principle applied at a famous Scottish teaching hospital which had finally accrued enough money to start its long-awaited rebuild. Funnily enough (or, to readers of this book – not surprisingly) the architects decided that Phase 1 would comprise a library, medical records and outpatients hall. This would allow them the maximum space for soaring ceilings etc – and perhaps even an atrium. The fact that the wards (where patients had to actually wash, undress and try to sleep) were falling apart mattered little. Anyway, Phase 1 got underway. The problem was that the scheme was far too grand to be labelled 'Outpatients' – and so the glass and concrete monstrosity was entitled 'Special Consultative Clinics'. Then the money ran out. Phase 1 was the only thing that got built. The reader will, despite the education given by this book, probably be surprised to learn of one of the many, many problems that beset the white elephant. The receptionists for the ENT Outpatients (now to be known as Special Consultative Clinic in Otorhinolaryngology) kept leaving and having to be replaced by women of sterner stuff. The reason for their departure? The typical Glaswegian would hit upon the word 'Special' when approaching the first clinic after the main entrance (hidden, in true modern building style). They were aggrieved to find when all they wanted was some treatment for a drippy willy[4] at the Special Clinic that they were being asked to have a hearing test.

The problem of changing names for no good reason is evidently not restricted to the UK. An ENT colleague from the Slovakian Republic[5] told us that the Health Service Managers in

---

[4]Medical term for 'urethral discharge' in male patients.

[5]We have no doubt that our readers (unlike President George W Bush, who actually thought that they were the same place!) will be well aware that the Slovakian Republic is an entirely different place and has a completely different language to the Republic of Slovenia.

Slovakia decided to call the ENT clinic the K.N.T. Clinic! To prevent patients confusing this with the gynaecology department, this was changed back to its old name.

Linguistic Barbarism

Languages other than dead languages (e.g. Latin, Sanskrit, Welsh) are alive in a sense that they are still growing, evolving and blossoming. The English language is particularly verbose and, according to the Guinness book of records, has the most words of all world languages – almost half a million.[6] Apart from new words, English changes in other, more subtle, ways. Some words change their meaning as time goes on, and sometimes their pronunciation. Indeed, one of the reasons cited by Doctor Johnson for writing his Dictionary was so that people would know how to spell 'waistcoat', the pronunciation of which had by 1755 become 'weskit'.[7] This evolution is, of course, part of the great joy of our own wonderful language. It gives us the privilege of using the richest, most colourful and expressive tongue in the world, full of nuance and innuendo.[8] A living

---

[6]It is doubtful, however, if any individual uses more than 60,000 words. Written English, in general, contains about 10,000 words, whilst spoken English (even among the better educated) has about 5,000.

[7]We are informed by our tailor, that nowadays many gentlemen (term here used in the wider sense) are reverting to the archaic pronunciation 'waste coat', which does of course have a completely different meaning.

[8]Indeed, your authors have here inadvertently used two words which exemplify the wider point. *Nuance* is French for colour or hue, and *innuendo* is a Latin gerund of the transitive verb *innuere*, to give a sign, hint or nod. There is no such word in Italian, as is often believed, and the plural therefore is never *innuendi*. Interestingly, Fowler suggests 'innuendos' whilst the *Oxford English Dictionary* prefers 'innuendoes'.

language is restless and unstable. No word is ever constant and immutable – nor ever has been. It was Doctor Johnson who derided the lexicographer who imagined

> that his dictionary can embalm his language and secure it from corruption and decay.

T S Eliot wrote:

> For last year's words belong to last year's language. And next year's await another voice.

For many years, certainly since the Middle Ages, the official language of medicine was Latin. Indeed, many doctors still write prescriptions out in that mother of languages. Greek was the language of Hippocrates[9], the father of medicine, and medicine borrows most of its terminology from these two classical languages.[10] 'Barbarism' is the linguistic term for a compound word made up of two different languages – and barbarisms make some classical scholars shudder! They consider that the roots of a word should either both be Latin, or both Greek and not a mixture – as in 'television'. This comes from *tele* (Greek for 'far off' or 'distant') and *video* (Latin for 'I see').[11] Homosexual, another barbarism derives from *homos* (Greek for 'the same')

---

[9]Actually, it was the Ionian dialect.

[10]For a very readable review of this, see Andrews E. *Medical Terminology*. Ann Med Hist 1928; 10:180–198.

[11]There were early critics who considered that television would never take off because its name was derived from bastard etymological origins!

while sexual is of Latin origin.[12] In Birchfield's brilliant book *The English Language*,[ii] we hear that

> compound words formed from elements drawn from two different languages give the kind of pain to a fastidious person that would be felt if a thistle were placed in the hands of a blindfolded man.

Birchfield goes on to say that

> Pretentiousness and officialdom are usually accompanied by an indefensible stretching out of syllables and an obscuration of meaning.

Whilst on the subject of pretentious officials, Sir Ernest Gowers, reviser of *Fowler's Modern English Usage* and author of *Plain Words*, pokes fun wonderfully at the jargon of officialdom and the solecisms of civil servants, trade union officials and managers. We have already noted that the Stasi appear to delight in an almost studied poor usage of English (see Chapter 3, Stark Naked Civil Servants) and that this can be likened to the traditional bad handwriting of doctors. Luckily, however, since they are most unlikely to ever be acquainted with classical languages, they are unlikely to offend their betters with anything more noisome than the 'word' HealthCare.

It was John Simons in *Paradigms Lost* who said that changes in language are born of ignorance. He considered that language is

---

[12]The word 'homosexual' is certainly a monster in the technical, mythological sense (the sense in which Wilde called hermaphrodites monsters) in as much as it consists of a Greek head on a Latin torso. It has, however, the merit not only of familiarity but also comprehensibility. (Brigid Brophy, *London Review of Books*, 21 April 1983, p8.)

'like a living organism that, like a live plant, sprouts new leaves and flowers', but continues that 'for the most part....changes out of ignorance'. Changing the meaning of words has, for whatever reason, been a feature of language since man began to speak, and some of these metamorphoses are fascinating. A good example of a non-medical, non-administrative word which has changed completely from its original meaning is *buxom*. This derives from the Anglo-Saxon verb *bugan* which means 'to bow'. The corresponding adjective, when it came into written English (around 1175) was *buhsom* and meant obliging, flexible or obedient. By the end of the sixteenth century, this had acquired three new meanings:

Unresisting – that is, directly from obedient.
Jolly or blithe [dare we say gay?]
Plump and comely.

As time has gone by only the plump and comely meaning has survived. Since the adjective is only ever applied to females (you just don't have buxom men!), what meant 'obedient' in the twelfth century has become 'voluptuous' or 'full-breasted' by the end of the twentieth. Perhaps the 'politically correct' term would be 'pectorally superior'.

The term politically correct (or even the abhorrent abbreviation PC) is itself a neologism which has only crept into our language over the past decade. One cynical definition of political correctness is that it is 'the incorrect use of language'. Perhaps this is what makes it particularly attractive to the Stasi.

The Stasi seem to be unhappy with their proper NHS title – they would like the name administrator changed to manager. One of us was actually told by a Chief Executive that she was not an administrator! The incident took place (as indeed most of the confrontations described herein) when your author had been summoned to a meeting with her and the Chairman of the Trust. The duel was set for 8 o'clock in the morning[13] and had been called because your author had appeared on local television[14]. This had occurred the previous week and had involved certain comments concerning the competence of the Stasi. This had not best pleased them. Your author (a tactful, patient, diplomatic sort of chap – as the perceptive reader will no doubt have deduced) listened for almost six minutes[15] then respectfully rose and started to leave the room, pointing out with sensitivity and finesse that he did not consider it proper or seemly for two Administrators (he did not use the term 'Stasi') to berate a consultant about what after all he considered to be his right of free speech.[16] His inquisitors asked him if he would please stay, but he declined.

Then, just as he was opening the door to leave, he was stopped in his tracks. The lady accountant (the CEO) said that before he went she wanted to set the record straight and that they were not

---

[13]Colleagues are advised only ever to attend interviews with the enemy at this hour, or even earlier. Doctors are used to getting out of bed at any time of day or night – Stasi certainly are not, and are therefore at an immediate disadvantage. Their initial reluctance to accede to attending a meeting this early is usually easily overcome. It must be pointed out that you are certainly willing to attend at this time, even if they are not! If they try to arrange a meeting during the working day, it is suggested that you grudgingly relent only after pointing out that you will write a personal letter to cancelled patients, identifying the Stasi by name and saying that this time had been insisted upon. It never fails!

[14]The mixed Greek-Latin origin of the word had not put him off.

[15]According to his tape recording. The absolute necessity of clandestine taping of all meetings has been already stressed, but bears repeating.

[16]Careful perusal of the tape confirmed that on this occasion he forbore to use the word impertinence and showed further exemplary self-restraint by not alluding to an officer having been summoned to the Sergeants' Mess.

Administrators! Your author was so shocked that he removed his spectacles! When he had composed himself, he asked for her definition of the word 'Administrator' and also enquired if either of them were familiar with the meaning of the word 'generic'. Rather than answer his questions, your author was told that it was he who was the great lover of dictionary definitions, not they (the perceptive reader will further realise that this remark, for once, contained a deal of truth). She seemed quite pleased with this snappy little riposte, presumably considering that for once she had managed to get the last word. Unabashed, your author promised he would look it up for her in the big dictionary as soon as the library opened. The time was now 0807. He went off to the canteen for another bacon sandwich; they just sat there, wondering what there was for them to do in the hospital at this time in the morning. As good as his word, the following morning, they both received this letter via the hospital post:[17]

Madam,
re. Definition of Administrator
Further to our meeting/confrontation this morning, I promised to look up the word 'administrator' in the dictionary: this I have now done.
The second of four definitions given in the *Concise Oxford Dictionary of Common English* (Clarendon, Oxford: R E Allen, 1988 8th ed, p16) is:
a person capable of administrating
You may now rest assured that I will never again refer to yourself or the Chairman as Administrators.
I have the great privilege to remain, ma'am &c &c.

---

[17]As did all the consultants at the hospital.

The Chairman wrote back saying that he thought the letter on the previous was not at all helpful.[iii]

Words Which Are Not Very Nice (Water Closets & Administrators)

The word 'water closet' is similar to the word 'administrator' in that there are certain people in society who would have us change that too. At the beginning of the twentieth century, the small room where one went to defaecate and urinate was known as a 'water closet'; this was because a 'closet' is a small room or cupboard, and the one in which one relieves oneself is fitted with piped water to flush away the effluent.[18] Evidently even the abbreviated term W.C. became unseemly and fell out of polite usage. It was replaced by the euphemism 'lavatory' which comes from the Latin *lavare* meaning to wash. Thus the word 'lavatory' (and also for that matter 'latrine') really means 'washing place'. Hence, the small room where one goes to pass water or open one's bowels is now known as a 'wash room'. This is reminiscent of the prissy hostess who might ask you if you wanted to wash your hands and then directs you to a room where the only water is in the WC (which has now come to mean the ceramic sanitary ware with the wooden seat, rather than the room in which it is situated). Although 'lavatories' are still used by a few diehards in the North of England, the 1950s brought the replacement words 'toilet' – this is French for 'hand towel'.[19] In its time, 'toilet' has been largely supplanted by 'loo' which is

---

[18]Similarly, an outside room with no water supply was called a 'privy' – from a private place.

[19]Interestingly, the authors' French dictionary (*Collins-Robert French-English Dictionary*, Glasgow: Harper Collins, 1994 4th ed p819) also lists *(Boucherie) toilette (de porc)* as lining of a pig's intestine wrapped around pieces of meat.

either a bad pun from water closet (or Water-loo) or is a direct derivative of *l'eau*. Either way, things have come full circle, or we are back where we started. The psychologists tell us that the reason why society changes certain words such as 'water closet' is that we don't feel comfortable with them. The concept of defaecation is far from attractive, so let us keep changing the name of the room where we do it. Bedsores too are particularly unattractive, often smelly, usually painful and invariably associated with poor nursing procedure. Surely it is far better to be a 'Tissue Viability Specialist' than a 'Bedsore Nurse'. Perhaps the same explanation obtains as to why this title has also been changed.

Other obvious examples of words which keep changing more rapidly than the slow evolution of language in general are epithets for ethnics. 'Coloured person', very acceptable to non-Caucasians ten years ago is now likely to cause offence. 'Black', by contrast, once forbidden, is now quite politically correct. One cannot help but wonder how the politically correct lobby deal with the thorny issue of Down's Syndrome. For many years they were always officially called Mongols. For one reason or another (dare we suggest racial arrogance by the whites) this name was considered degrading. Following this line of reasoning, then a vast number of the world's population are not quite up to scratch[20] – and this itself may then be considered racist.

All this is a sign of how society is getting prissier. All doctors

---

[20]This is a dog fighting term (one of your authors used to keep bull terriers) – the scratch is the start-line (like the oche in darts). Before the start of the fight, the dogs stand at this line growling, pulling, scratching and straining to get at their opponent. If a dog does not fancy his chance, then he doesn't come up to scratch. The reader will note that this information is not found in many books!

know that *orchis* is Greek for *testis* (which is Latin for 'witness') and there is no comparable word in English (at least not in polite usage). Orchidectomy then means surgical removal of the testicle, and 'Ballockworts'[iv] was the Middle English name for orchid plants.[21] Mind you, if you look at the tubers of orchids, you will readily appreciate how they got their name.

Ignorance is the Mother of Impudence[22]

Delusions of grandeur and its association with the later forms of that hideous disease syphilis have been explored when talking about the Stasi in Chapter 1. An impertinence which sadly is becoming commonplace in hospitals is the use of the salutation 'Dear Colleague', when administration is writing to doctors. One of us has to admit that this particular discourtesy when written by accountants used to irritate him so intensely that his response to it led first of all to a lot of acrimonious correspondence between him and the lady CEO but eventually to his winning an award.[23]

The correct procedure, of course, when a consultant receives any letter addressed in this manner is either to consign it

---

[21]'Shit' is another vulgarism which has fallen out of polite usage. It was used in old medical texts. Chaucer too often used it, and in Caxton's *Aesops Fables* we are told, 'I dide shyte tre grete toordes'. This points out in fact that 'shite' should strictly be used as a verb, and the word shit reserved for substantive (noun) usage.

[22]As always, your authors wish to remain fair and objective, and this proverb from Bohn's 1855 *Handbook of Proverbs* makes the charitable assumption that some Stasi and hospital executives know no better; cf. the Christian admonition, 'Forgive them, for they know not what they do.'

[23]He has come to think this is the only sort of award he will ever get. The actual award was from the prestigious Mackenzie Society of London which awarded him its medal in 1997 for a presentation of his collated letters to the Chief Executive.

immediately to the wastepaper basket (on the irrebuttable assumption it has reached the wrong addressee) or to return it to the sender marked 'Apologies – Opened in Error – addressed to Colleague'. This latter is precisely what was done when such a letter was received by your author (and the other consultants at the hospital where he worked at the time) from the lady CEO.[v] Nonetheless, a second identical missive soon arrived on your author's desk and this was consigned straightway to the bin! After a telephone call from the CEO's secretary demanding a reason for your author's failure to respond, he wrote a formal letter pointing out the dictionary definition of colleague, viz:

> colleague n. fr. Fr. *collègue* from. Lat *collega* 'one chosen at the same time as another; associate' from col- & leg-, 'pick out, select' &c. a. One associated with another or others in any occupation esp. of an official character; thus a minister of the Crown is a colleague of the other ministers, or professor at a university is the colleague of other professors at the same university and so on, and one will speak of another as my colleague so-and-so; b. applied also to persons of the same profession though otherwise in no way connected, e.g. a London surgeon might speak of Edinburgh surgeons as colleagues. Less commonly used of persons associated in purely commercial pursuits.[vi]

He then went on to point out in fairly clear terms:

You are therefore not my colleague, nor a colleague of any of the consultant medical staff at this hospital (as far as I know, none of my colleagues are accountants).

After a diplomatic request that 'this discourteous lack of protocol' should not be repeated, the letter concluded

> I have the great honour to remain, ma'am, your most obedient servant but not your colleague![vii]

Before the next joust could take place, however, she wrote to him instructing him, in effect, not to circulate any more letters to the other consultants. She told him that he must not misuse Trust resources. In fact, she wrote:

> Without being prescriptive [*sic*] this includes secretarial time and other resources spent in circulating correspondence of little relevance to at least some of the recipients.[viii]

In response to this directive, your author wrote (and, of course, sent copies to all his colleagues) the following:

> At the risk of seeming pedantic about the correct use of English (nay, perish the thought!) may I point out that when you say 'without being prescriptive...' (vide supra), I and most of the colleagues to whom I have shown your letter think perhaps you mean 'proscriptive'. Those of us who were lucky enough to have had a classical education will be aware of the interesting etymology of the word, and in Roman history,

---

[24]*Proscriptio* or possibly 'proscription' refers in Roman history particularly to the wholesale proscriptions of the dictator Sulla (138–78 BC) who led a reign of terror in Rome and Italy, drawing up long lists of enemies to be executed. According to Smith: 'No one was safe; for Sulla gratified his friends by placing in the fatal lists their personal enemies or those who property was coveted' (Smith W. *Smaller Classical Dictionary London*: Murray, 20th Ed p404.) Notwithstanding, Sulla was a well-educated man with a great love of beauty, literature and the liberal arts.

proscription[24] was publication of a list of names of persons condemned to banishment or death. A mnemonic you could perhaps use in future is that doctors prescribe but hospital Administrators proscribe.[ix]

A formal meeting did eventually take place at which your author was threatened with disciplinary action if he used Trust resources to send copies of his letters to the CEO to other consultants! He therefore graciously conceded the point and followed the simple expedient of having future epistles copied on a friend's photocopier and delivering them to his colleagues by hand, admonishing them on receipt under no circumstances to read them until they got out of the hospital.

Soon afterwards the lady resigned!

The reader may be very interested to know that the GMC's definitive ruling on the colleague matter.[x] In order, principally to set the poor lady's mind at rest, and believing that she was very concerned about her correct usage of English in general and this word colleague in particular, your author wrote[25] to the president of the GMC for clarification once and for all on this important matter. A reply came promptly, and if he had read paragraph 20 of their booklet 'Good Medical Practice,' he would already have known the answer: 'Colleague clearly refers to a registered medical practitioner.'

He had to admit that this final word on the subject was more restrictive than he had imagined. Two thoughts sprang to mind. Was he now to consider foreign doctors and housemen[26]

---

[25]Using his own writing paper, envelope and stamp.

[26]Strictly speaking, housemen i.e. doctors immediately after qualification in their first year of work (US: interns) are still under the auspices of the medical school. They do not register until after one probationary year and only then subject to a good report.

colleagues (he had always done so, and also for that matter medical students[27]). The second thought was cynical and perhaps unworthy of him. Did the GMC have a vested interest in this *clear* definition? Whilst musing on this he started to worry if he himself had paid his annual retention fee (for if he had forgotten, not only would he be unable to practise legally, but he himself would have no colleagues!).

Words Only To Conceal[28]

The reader has seen how the English language is constantly evolving and slowly changing, and how indeed we English are the richer for it. The concept of political correctness, which we have defined as 'the incorrect use of English' has been explored as a way that insidious elements of society inimical to tradition have used our wonderful tongue and tried to accelerate the slow evolution of our language to a whirlwind speed for radical political motives.

The Stasi have made use of this trend to change words for their own ulterior objectives. In an attempt to emasculate doctors they have tried to change the meaning of the word 'colleague' so that it includes themselves. Because the term 'Administrator' has become so odious to people who actually work in hospitals, it has been supplanted by the epithet 'Manager' in the vain hope that people will think they are not the same thing! They probably

---

[27]Your other author was once told by a kindly old physician 'What I am, you will be; what you are, I was.' It seems to encapsulate the bond nicely.

[28]The full quote is from Voltaire: '*Ils ne servent de la pensée que pour autoriser leurs injustices, et n'emploient les paroles que pour déguiser leurs pensées.*' For the benefit of any Stasi who have reached this penultimate chapter, the authors tender not only hearty congratulations but a translation: 'Men use thought only to justify their misdeeds, and words only to conceal their thought.'

do not even know that they are now known as 'Stasi' (and even if they do they probably don't know what it alludes to.)

In some hospitals they have issued directives about the revised use of the word 'committee'. A Drug & Therapeutics Committee had been meeting for years to discuss topics on such matters as policies concerning the use of narcotic drugs on hospital patients, and debating the adoption of new antibiotics or other recently developed drugs in the hospital pharmacy. Most lay people would, your authors believe, consider this important. This committee was informed a few years ago, however, that the Stasi didn't mind them continuing in this work, but it would no longer be possible for them to be considered a 'committee'. In future this word was only to be used for bodies reporting directly to the Chief Executive. The committee members, mainly consultants and pharmacists thought that this was some sort of joke, but were quickly assured that this was not the case. So they re-christened themselves the Drugs & Therapeutics Dining Club.

The word which has changed in meaning more than any other, however, is 'Trust'. What is now called a Trust used once to be called an Authority. That was in the old days of plain speaking. One knew where one was with an authority. The definition is: 'the right to command and enforce obedience'. It is paradoxical that as Hospital Authorities have become more commanding and forceful, and in the case of West Midlands, draconian (see the next chapter) they have changed their name to 'Trust'. One definition of the word Trust is 'a firm conviction in one's reliability, integrity and honour.'

Isn't it strange how, in a comparatively short space of time, a word has now become the complete opposite, the absolute antithesis of its former meaning. But, there again, in the dictionary, which the father of one of your authors used to carry in his satchel every day to school, the word 'gay' is defined as 'merry, sportive; brilliant; charming, attractive'![xi]

We must, of course, guard against the dangers of oversimplification, as exemplified by one of the doctors in Richard Dooling's *Critical Care* when trying to explain the complexities of chemotherapy:

> We are going to give you and the tumours a lot of poison and see which one of you dies first. Sometimes that works. Since you're so much bigger than the tumours, you've got a better chance of surviving.[xii]

We must also guard against the well-meaning 'reformer' – the following appeared in the journal *The Practising Midwife*:

> Delivery is a word that Mary has learnt not to use in relation to childbirth – 'letters are delivered, babies are born'. Mary believes that the language we use around childbirth has an important, if subtle, impact on our attitudes and approach. We should use language carefully, being sure to avoid words which are disrespectful, disempowering or depersonalising.[xiii]

One of the authors wrote the following letter to the editor, Jilly Rosser MEd RM Midwifery Consultant[29]:

> Letter to the Editor – Empowerment through English?
> I think the aims of Mary in trying to avoid language which is disrespectful, disempowering or depersonalising (Editorial

---

[29]Note the use of the word 'consultant'.

The Practising Midwife 1998; 1(7):45) are praiseworthy. In banning the word 'delivery', I believe she has gone too far. Words can be appropriate – or wilfully misinterpreted; an example might be 'practising'. We all know that 'practice makes perfect', it is just a 'practice shot' – it does not harm our use of the word to describe our work (or this journal!).

The consequence of abolishing 'delivery' will be the birth of a new verb 'birthing', along the lines of 'has this mother birthed yet? Will you help with this birthing?' I do not feel that this is progress.

Amazingly enough, the letter was published!

We should not be critical of all words, though. 'Collaboration' is, of course, a Good Thing. We are all members of a team. Except at weekends and during the night. The team seems to contract somewhat then.

CHAPTER 8

DISCIPLINING HOSPITAL DOCTORS IN THE NATIONAL HEALTH SERVICE

Despite the authors' attempts to approach the present confrontation bedevilling the NHS with humour and common sense, it should be said that it has already reached serious levels of incipient totalitarianism, as the reader will see from Dr Tomlin's following chapter on the current abuses of disciplinary procedures. 'Shroud waving' is a dismissive term invented by the Stasi for professional warnings of hazards to patients that are unpalatable (i.e. have cost implications). The suppression of criticism, muzzling the professions, and institutional disregard of the law, are well-known symptoms to those familiar with the history of the evolution of Nazi Germany and Soviet Russia, to name but two. It is devoutly to be hoped that the disease can be fought.

You may think we are exaggerating. Well, consider this, which formed part of an opening address Peter gave to the West London Medical-Chirurgical Society, November 2002, which we paraphrase here:

Imagine an industrial process, which when used made half the workers ill, some seriously, and caused a 2% mortality. Imagine that the management knew all about it (and have known so for years) and do nothing about it. Neither does the Government. There would be a public outcry![i]

Gentlemanly Conduct[1]

Apart from the disciplinary procedures in the NHS, doctors are subject to two other codes of conduct:

- that embedded in the criminal code, and to which all citizens are subject
- that exercised by the General Medical Council (GMC).

The GMC concerns itself with ethical and professional conduct, fitness to practise and professional standards of competence. As we have previously outlined, in the past there was also the Medical Superintendent. This was usually a very senior doctor chosen by medical peers. In the event of a dispute between colleagues (for example about operating times, beds or equipment), he would do the equivalent of taking them round the back of the bicycle shed and banging their heads together. There are two important points, which need to be made, even at this early stage of the chapter:

- the Medical Superintendent was respected
- there was no attempt at public humiliation.

---

[i]It was Thomas Arnold (1795–1842), the famous headmaster of Rugby School who in his Address to his Scholars said: 'What we must look for here is, first, religious and moral principles; secondly, gentlemanly conduct; thirdly, intellectual ability.'

Doctors provided the ethos behind the hospitals. The overwhelming majority were (and probably still are!) severely workaholic; this was, and still is, we believe, inculcated in their training. Their professionalism drove them to put the patients first, before themselves, their families or their friends. They jeopardized not only their social life, but, especially in days when infectious diseases were common, their own health as well.

Nurses have also shared this professionalism – but with one exception. This is time management. It dates back to Florence Nightingale, who held that nurses must work regular shifts. This tradition persists to this day. Of course, many nurses do have to work over – and the concept of 'time owing' covers this. It is not a phrase found in medical circles, where, until very recently, shift work was unknown. The medical profession has always been of the opinion that the job ends when the work is finished. This ethic that the patient comes first, before family commitments, and certainly well ahead of any duty to the employer, is anathema to the Stasi. To them, the patients are mere ciphers.

Of course, there used to be respect and loyalty to the hospital when it was obvious that the institution was doing everything it could for the patients and that all workers were pulling together (and in the same direction). Respect and loyalty were reciprocated – something the Americans would probably call a 'two-way street', owing to the difficulty they have with words of more than one syllable. But we digress (again).

Things were not always perfect, and it is well known that there was gross exploitation, some of which persists. It was not uncommon to have virtually no time off during a six-month house job. Marriage was frowned on, as were extra-curricular activities. Junior house staff not only worked but also lived in the hospital, and for a very low salary compared with their schoolmates who had left university for other professions. Why did they put up with it? Probably for two reasons – they expected light at the end of the tunnel, and they saw their seniors also working hard for their patients. They also saw their seniors were respected members of a respected profession, and this was something that they aspired to.

Doctors have always squabbled amongst themselves, and this is not surprising. They are trained to lead, accept responsibility for their actions, and shape events. It has become rather a 'catch-phrase' now, but they have been trained to be the patient's advocate. The patient comes to the physician with a medical problem, for which he seeks relief. A practitioner who does not show enterprise and initiative, who does not seek improved facilities and a fair share of the financial cake for his patients would be considered not to be using his training or doing his job properly. Once agreements were struck, they were adhered to, as there was mutual respect. It was not always the case that those who shouted the loudest got the most; each had gone through the same basic training and shared the same basic professional ethics.

Three things happened in the late 1940s to change this. First, the war ended, the armed forces returned to civilian life, and many young doctors returned to claim the hospital jobs they had left when they joined up at the beginning of the war. These posts had been guaranteed for them at the end of hostilities. Some had gone to war a very short time after qualification, but returned as very experienced practitioners. Second, the NHS was established. Hospital treatment was no longer means-tested and became unrestrictedly free to all. This exposed an unmet need, and later a growing demand, in society – patients flocked to the hospitals. Third, consultants in voluntary hospitals received a salary for the first time, but were able to continue the private practice that had hitherto supported them only in the wealthier centres.

The relatively few senior doctors in post were able, indeed, had to, delegate the extra work to their experienced juniors, and the senior who did not teach, or had no reputation, would formerly have had few juniors. With the inevitable expansion of the work of the hospitals, governments, reluctant to fund increases in expensive consultants, disproportionately increased the numbers of cheaper junior posts. The result was a glut of fully trained specialists queuing for too few consultant posts. This led to an emigration brain drain in the late 1950s and early 1960s. So-called training posts became filled with permanently junior immigrant doctors and the hospital service was for many years sustained on a shoestring budget by the dedication of a generation of doctors and nurses who had lived through the war and were accustomed to self-sacrifice in a humanitarian cause.

Nevertheless, the bill for this initial election vote-winner became a political headache to successive governments who have been unprepared to invest adequate amounts of money into it. Public dissatisfaction was seen to be aggravated by doctors and nurses representing the needs of their patients, who (worse!) were themselves seen to have more faith in the professions than in the government propaganda. The multiple reorganisations of the NHS have largely been clumsy attempts to curb expenditure while avoiding electoral backlash by a combination of double-talk and stifling informed criticism. In the case of doctors and nurses this has been pursued by systematically denigrating the professions in the eyes of the public, removing them from effective authority in the hospitals, and trying to impose a bureaucratic dictatorship. Any reader with experience in the teaching profession will recognise the pattern.

The Discipline System in Theory

In 1961, the Stasi produced their first major disciplinary code, HM 61 112. This was a circular produced by Her Majesty's Stationery Office and distributed to all health authorities; it has been the mainstay of all disciplinary procedures against doctors since then. It classifies offences into one of three categories:

- Professional Incompetence (e.g. making a clinical mistake)
- Professional Misconduct (e.g. refusing to visit a sick person)
- Personal Misconduct (e.g. armed robbery)

Legally, the first two categories have always been the responsibility of the GMC. The Stasi have tried to ride roughshod over this, proclaiming that this was merely a system of doctors banding together to cover up their mistakes whilst protecting each other. The basis of a profession (such as medicine, law etc) is self-regulation, and, at least for the time being, Parliament seems content with this. The Stasi do not form a profession: indeed this would be an oxymoron[2]. They can never therefore have a professional body such as the GMC (called the General Management Council) to oversee them; there is no offence of Managerial Incompetence or Managerial Misconduct; there are no Fitness to Manage Committees; there is no Management Governance. There are certainly daily examples of Management

---

[2]'Oxymoron' is a linguistic term for the bringing together of two opposites or the combining in one expression of two terms that are ordinarily contradictory. It is from the Greek for 'sharp-witted' (oxos) and 'dullard' (moron). It is most often used in poetry (e.g. 'His honour, rooted in dishonour stood.' Tennyson 'Lancelot and Elaine'; 'Our final hope is flat despair.' Milton. 'Paradise Lost.'; 'Loveliness... is when unadorn'd, adorn'd the most.' Thomson, 'Autumn') It can also be used humorously (e.g. 'A truthful twenty-first-century century politician'; 'a cheerful pessimist'; 'harmonious discord'; 'professional hospital Stasi' etc).

Negligence but it does not have an associated disciplinary code. It is perhaps not surprising that the Stasi resent the GMC and try to override its actions. As the reader will see, such attempts serve neither the patient nor taxpayer well – and the doctors not at all.

I'll Be The Judge; I'll Be The Jury[3]

It will be seen that, in usurping disciplinary powers, the Stasi have become rather like vigilantes, unconcerned about the harm they may cause to innocent victims who are tried and lynched by a mob acting outside the due processes of law and natural justice.

Professional incompetence was to be judged by a panel of medical practitioners[4], of whom only one need be a member of the accused doctor's specialty. Theoretically, this could lead to the absurd situation where physicians could be asked to pronounce on the technical competence of surgeons or anaesthetists, or any other combination. More than anything else, this exposed the level of ignorance among the administration. The disciplinary panel is chosen in part from nominees from the profession, and in part from people chosen by the accusing health authority. It is understood that it tends to be formed of people attuned to the authority's way of thinking – those who 'know what is required'. Although such a panel would contain doctors, they would be in a minority, not of the accused's specialty and probably sympathetic to the authority. The code actually states that the laymen were to

---

[3]The reader may have come to the justifiable conclusion that this whole chapter is from *Alice in Wonderland*! It is not, but we have borrowed this heading from Lewis Carroll's (*Alice's Adventures In Wonderland*, Chapter 3). Alice daydreams:
'I'll be the Judge, I'll be the Jury,'
said cunning old Fury:
'I'll try the whole case, and condemn you to death.'

[4]Later adjusted so that the chairman (or chair!) was a senior legally-qualified layman.

be chosen by the prosecuting health authority! This is not only contrary to the rules of natural justice, but also expressly against the rules of *Habeas Corpus* and the Convention of Human Rights. Even if the prosecuting authority did not nominate its own sycophantic lackeys, the nominees could never be considered wholly impartial.

The third in the list of offences, Personal Misconduct, was to be judged by the Stasi themselves. For this, they have available the same system used for all grades of hospital staff.

It can be seen that the Stasi can fill every role in such kangaroo courts except that of the accused. They are accusers, investigators, prosecutors, judge, jury and appeal court. With such a system, something not out of place in a totalitarian state, one would think that justice would, if not fair, at least be speedy, cheap and efficient! Of course, it is none of these things, and especially, it is not fair.

Better Sit Idle Than Work For No Pay[5]

In all cases, a guilty verdict spells dismissal from work; since the NHS is virtually a monopoly employer, this means the end of paid employment. It is hardly possible to transfer geographical locations since dismissal on a disciplinary charge effectively means being blacklisted. The accused becomes an economic exile. Sending people into exile was once the prerogative of kings and judges; to this we must now add hospital administrators supported by amateur ad hoc committees accountable to no one!

This whole process is contrary not only to the European Convention but also the United Nations Universal Declaration of Human Rights. There was a right of appeal to the Secretary of

---

[5]Seventeenth-century proverb.

State. He had it in his power to convene an Appeal Panel to reconsider the case. However, the Secretary of State was not bound to accept the findings of the Appeal Panel. This situation (which the reader might find reminds him of something somewhere between the operettas of Gilbert and Sullivan and the writings of Kafka) can, and indeed has, resulted in the doctor being found innocent of the charges on appeal – but then nobody taking any notice of the verdict.

Pay Without Work[6]

A problem inherent in HM 61 112 is that there is no time limit on how long a doctor might be suspended from the hospital. Fortunately, no Stasi has yet been stupid enough to deny a doctor admission to hospital as a patient – though this has been used as an excuse to get rid of him by seeking to impose early retirement on the grounds of ill health! Because of this lack of time limit, a doctor might be deprived of his professional liberty for years. This might even be without any charge being brought. Since a suspended doctor is usually on full pay (they haven't been able to stop that yet), there is consequently a considerable cost to the taxpayer. Normally (in the outside world, where the rules of law apply), no person can be deprived of a civil liberty for more than a very limited amount of time (measured in hours) without the approval of the courts, no matter how serious the charge – and there has to be a charge.

The longest cases of suspension of doctors were two of about equal length. Both were prevented from practising their

---

[6]Over 200 years before the strange concept of 'Suspension on Full Pay', Dr Samuel Johnson defined Pension in his dictionary as, 'Pay given to a state hireling for treason to his country.'

profession for over ten years (without charge being brought against them, and on full pay). It is perhaps significant that they were both female. The prolonged suspension of one of them eventually resulted in the Chief Executive of the Health Service being severely admonished by the Public Accounts Committee in the House of Commons. This certainly must have been unpleasant, but it did not actually personally cost him a penny. To be fair, he had never been involved in the suspension, but had inherited it from his predecessor. There followed a very critical House of Commons report on the maladministration involved.

In 1990, as a result of pressure generated by various sectors of the profession, the disciplinary code was revised, the revisions being published in a health circular HC90/9. The most important change was the introduction of time limits for suspension, although, amazingly, this did not include suspension without charge! It also denied the right of appeal to the Secretary of State in cases of personal misconduct (which were a waste of time anyway, as they were unlikely to be upheld *even if successful*). Another key instruction in HC90/9 was that more openness should be practised and that justice should be seen to be done.

Health authorities have, for the most part, ignored HC90/9. Despite specific instruction to the contrary, they continue to hold their unlawful hearings and tribunals behind closed doors and there is little evidence that their make up is unbiased.[ii] The contrast with the very public GMC disciplinary hearings speaks volumes. The only reason for holding disciplinary hearings in secret is to allow prejudice, malice and lies to fester. Health authorities are afraid to let the public see what is going on or what constitutes their 'justice'.

Another important feature of HC90/9 was the introduction of

the concept of lesser charges being dealt with rather more efficiency, but without the sanction of dismissal. For such cases, a two-man team would be asked to investigate. There was no right of cross-examination and witnesses could even be interviewed in secret. The accused need not know who was making the allegations and was denied any chance of challenging their truthfulness. After such a 'trial', the 'verdict' was conveyed to the local Chief Executive of the Hospital Trust. A disturbing trend is after having had such a trial, and having agreed initially that the alleged offences were minor, such an executive might then decide that the accused doctor should go through the full rigours of the disciplinary code (including suspension and dismissal) *for the same offence.*

In October 1994, the Department of Health published another revision, HSG 94/49 – this time a 'Guide Line'. It states:

> Occasionally it is necessary to suspend a medical practitioner. However, misuse of this power can result in individual injustice and major waste of public money. Recent cases have highlighted that this leads to corrosion of public confidence in the NHS.

It lays down specific guidelines to time limits for suspension which should be kept to 'an absolute minimum in all cases'. A further document from the BMA's Central Consultants and Specialists Committee (CCSC) and the NHS Confederation in May 1997 emphasised the need for time limits. In October 1998, the CCSC Chairman, Dr Peter Hawker said, 'The guidelines are being flouted'.[iii] That same month, it was announced in *Hospital Doctor* that the number of suspended consultants had risen tenfold since the beginning of the year and was now at record levels. Dr

Bernard Charnley, a histopathologist suspended by the North Glamorgan Trust some four years previously said that the guidance was not worth the paper it was written on and that there was no procedure for enforcing the recommendations. All the Department of Health requires when the time limits are overshot is simply to be informed. That is all! In stark contrast to this, common criminals and even suspected terrorists cannot be held except under very special circumstances and for a set limited time only.

The Disciplinary System in Practice

Suspensions are supposed to be for serious matters only, according to HM61/112. This seems reasonable. But what constitutes a 'serious matter'? It is up to the Stasi to decide. One practitioner was suspended for writing the ward sister a prescription – to save her a visit to her doctor's surgery. This very act is allowed in other hospitals where it is recognised that everybody's time and effort are saved. Another physician was suspended because he overstayed his annual leave (which he had taken on an emergency basis) by four days. The authority refused to acknowledge that the reason for this was that his father was dying. The extra four days were to organise and attend his funeral. There are many examples, each showing that a malicious person can always find some pretext or other to further his nefarious ends.

Sometimes it is not so much malice as sheer incompetence. A doctor was suspended following claims that he had filled in the wrong forms concerning the Mental Health Act. It took the Stasi nine months to admit their error and acknowledge that the doctor had been right. Another doctor was suspended for refusing on safety grounds to re-sheathe used hypodermic needles. Soon, but not soon enough to prevent his dismissal and the subsequent ruining of his career, the authority issued a ruling that staff were not to re-sheathe the needles, owing to the health risk.

Sometimes it is neither malice nor incompetence. A consultant orthopaedic surgeon was ordered by the Chief Executive to start using some new hip prostheses, which had been bought cheaply in a job lot. He had previously rejected the choice on the grounds of patient safety. He was duly suspended. It eventually transpired that his fears were well grounded, for many patients who had had them inserted had to have them removed – at great cost and not a little danger. No action was taken against the Stasi.

We Will Get You – One Way Or Another

In the same way that Blacklegs[7] were ostracized by Trade Unionists in the 1950s, before the Industrial Relations Act, so some suspended doctors are 'sent to Coventry'[8] by the other hospital workers. One might reasonably presume that malicious rumours are spread by the Stasi (since they are often the only ones who know the reason for the suspension!).

A very bizarre aspect of the whole process is the lockout – this

---

[7] These were originally swindlers, especially in cards and at race meetings. The term later came to be used for those who worked for less than union wages.

[8] This term is interesting in its derivation. Brewer in his 1894 *Dictionary of Phrase & Fable* gives the meaning: 'To let him live and move and have his being with you, but pay no more heed to him than to the idle winds which regard you not.' *Chambers's Cyclopaedia* would have us believe that it derives from the citizens there having such a dislike of the Roman soldiery that a woman seen speaking to one was instantly tabooed; hence when a soldier was sent to Coventry, he was cut off from all social intercourse.

Hutton's *History of Birmingham*, however, gives the later and more obscure explanation that since Coventry was a Parliamentary stronghold during the Civil War, troublesome and refractory Royalists were sent there for safe custody.

is when a suspended doctor is effectively exiled from the hospital. The authorities have no legal right whatsoever to enforce this lockout unless it has already been agreed in the contract of employment. In fact, when such exclusion denies the opportunity to collect evidence, that is itself a serious breach of the disciplinary codes. Hospitals are public places and one has to wonder how the banishment has ever been enforced. It must be a measure of how intimidated the poor suspended doctor must have felt that he took any notice of the despotic Stasi who excluded him. One has to suppose that suspended practitioners are so fearful for their own future that they accede to this illegal and unreasonable demand. What after all can the authority do to keep the doctor out if he chooses to challenge their authority and visit the hospital? The police would certainly never get involved, and the hospital security guards could not physically manhandle any peaceful doctor without committing assault. Your authors would certainly hope that none of their readers is ever suspended, but if (perish the thought!) they ever are, it is suggested that they totally ignore this illicit lockout, and visit the hospital every day. Even if they are not able to collate their counter-evidence (because one assumes that they will not have been told the charges!) at least they can go and sit quietly in the public areas wearing something bright[9] – the foyer, WRVS or League of Friends Coffee Bars. They can visit as many inpatients as possible, and take lunch in the medical dining room (if it still exists) on a daily basis.

Suspended doctors, on the whole, have not challenged this exclusion and there are some terrible stories of how this tyranny

---

[9]One of those DayGlo tabards marked 'Doctor' which St John doctors wear at road traffic accidents might be considered overdoing it.

has affected some very vulnerable doctors. An extreme example was the case of a doctor who was himself admitted to the intensive care unit of the hospital as a patient. He was told to remove himself 'as he was an embarrassment to the hospital'. Another doctor was prevented from visiting his dying wife. In a third case, the wife appealed to the Community Health Council that her husband should have visiting rights in the event of her illness worsening. By the time this permission came, she was dead.

These are all recorded cases – they are not made up!

Even the most jaundiced, anti-medical reader would surely concede that suspended doctors should be afforded at least those rights extended to convicted criminals and terrorists.

For those lucky readers who have managed to live this long without involving themselves unduly with the law, we will reiterate that it is one of the great cornerstones of English law that an accused person must be presumed innocent until proven otherwise 'beyond any reasonable doubt'. The Stasi claim that this exile, which they euphemistically choose to call 'exclusion' rather than 'suspension' does not imply guilt and is a neutral act. If this is so, then such a 'neutral exile' must be as common as a ballet dancer's wife! Recently the House of Lords[10] pronounced that suspensions are clearly not a neutral act. In the House of Commons[11], no less a person than the Secretary of State for

---

[10]Perhaps those unfamiliar with the British parliamentary system can be forgiven for failing to appreciate that the House of Lords is the Highest Court (Supreme Judiciary) in the United Kingdom of Great Britain and Northern Ireland. Failure to know this cannot however be given as an excuse by the Stasi.

[11]The House of Commons is the Lower house of the Parliament of the United Kingdom. Parliament also includes the Sovereign and the Upper house, the House of Lords; the House of Commons is the dominant branch.

Health has also said that suspension is not a neutral act. In fact he went so far as to describe it as 'a deeply hostile act.'(Milburn 1995)[iv] At the time, he was supported in this description by Dr Liam Donaldson, later to become the Chief Medical Officer.[v] This attack on suspensions, however, was made when neither of them were attached to the Department of Health. The Secretary of State for Health was on the Public Accounts Committee at the time and Dr Donaldson was not yet CMO. Since they joined the DoH, for some reason they seem to have lost interest in this subject. Our readers will not be too surprised that the Stasi too have decided to ignore the ruling of the highest court in the land and in June 2007, the front page of a regional newspaper reassured its readers:

> The Trust stresses that suspension is a neutral act, taken in accordance with procedures, which allows time for a full, objective investigation of the complaint.[vi]

During the 'lockout', there is commonly a campaign of character assassination during which opinions are canvassed in a trawl for adverse statements. There need be no pretence of a scientific survey – things that support the doctor's case can simply be discarded! In one case, the Stasi had not even the wit to keep his mouth shut, simply exclaiming: 'I cannot use these: they favour Doctor X.'[12]

The supporting documents were destroyed. It is in fact sometimes surprising that such support is forthcoming, for there are plenty of ways of intimidating juniors into providing what is required. Another weapon in their armoury is the leaking of

---

[12]Not his real name.

words to the media such as 'suspension is because these are very serious matters which must be looked into', amid claims about a large dossier being compiled. As it is the Stasi who do the looking and compiling, little can be said to the contrary.[13] All this makes nonsense of the so-called neutrality of suspension.

In 1998, a fresh-faced youth called Stephen Thornton, apparently the Chief Executive of the NHS Confederation, said:

Remember that suspension is not a punishment. Suspension needs to be seen in the context of what is in the best interest of the patients [Authors' Note: It is of course well-known to all, and especially to the reader who has read so far, that the Stasi think of little else but the welfare of the patient!] and I think that suspensions of doctors need to be seen in the same way as suspensions of any other members of staff. It is interesting that it is only medical staff where we have these problems ... my question is: does this root back to the particularly special status that medical staff has? They cannot have their cake and eat it.[vii]

To this, the authors would say that it is certainly very reassuring to know that this sapling Chief Executive accords a 'particular special status' to doctors.

A recently noted development has been the attempt to impose a form of house arrest. Not only has the doctor been banished from his place of work, but told to remain at home close by a telephone. It is difficult to see how such a form of house arrest

---

[13]When Jonathan Swift wrote about 'the most pernicious race of odious little vermin that nature ever suffered to crawl upon the surface of the earth' (*Gulliver's Travels*, 1726), he was not referring to hospital administrators.

can be considered neutral. It is certainly unenforceable in law, and in fact, the law has come to the aid of many doctors hounded from their posts and then 'reinstated'. A suspended doctor has successfully sued (and won considerable damages) for the way he had been treated, and in particular, for the way in which he had been 'summoned' back to work. The judge's ruling was that: 'After being treated so badly a consultant is entitled to time to consider whether a return to work at all is reasonable.'

This was because following such an affair, the natural trust and confidence that must exist between employer and employee had been undermined – the suspended doctor was entitled to take as long as he liked (within reason)[14] in deciding whether ever to work again with such an untrustworthy employer.

Court Protection And *Habeas Corpus*[15]

Habeas corpus is a safeguard in English Law against wrongful imprisonment. There is apparently no equivalent for those doctors deprived of their professional liberty. One of the consequences of *Habeas Corpus* is that the periods of deprivation of liberty are strictly defined, and the accusers must go back to the court if they require more time. They will be called

---

[14]'Within reason' is one of those beautiful legal phrases that make lawyers rich.

[15]*Habeas corpus* is an important legal principle defined as a provision of *Magna Carta* and added to in the reign of Charles II. The original act essentially provided:
1. that any man taken to prison can insist that his accusers shall take him bodily before a judge and state the why and wherefore of his detention; *habeas corpus* – you (the accusers) are to produce the body (before the judge);
2. that every person accused of a crime shall be tried by twelve impartial men, and not by a goverment agent or nominee;
3. no prisoner shall be tried more than once on the same charge;
4. every prisoner may insist on being examined within twenty days of his arrest.

upon to justify their request. It is plain to see that the disciplinary code needs something similar.

Appeal to the courts for natural justice has proved useless. On one occasion, a doctor (after suspension of a year) appealed to the court for an explanation as to why he had been suspended. The hospital authority claimed that it had a dossier of hundreds of cases to go through. The fact was that they were trawling through the entire medical records of his career in a vain attempt to find some evidence on which to justify themselves. They found nothing. The problem was that the judge set them no time limit, but simply allowed them to get on with it. It was only after two and a half years that the Authority withdrew all its allegations of wrongdoing.

A few years ago, a doctor won his appeal to the Secretary of State and therefore should have been reinstated. Nevertheless, the Authority refused to do so. He returned to court and won a judgement that he 'should be found a job according to the contractually agreed rules'. The administration flouted the court order, and the Secretary of State then tergiversated and confirmed the dismissal. Once again, the doctor returned to the courts. The judge now said, in effect, that a reinstatement could not be ordered and that our poor supplicant had 'reached the end of the line'. He had not. He went to the European Court of Human Rights – and won.

As briefly mentioned earlier, another nasty little ploy which the unscrupulous can resort to is that of 'shroud waving'. They claim that they are acting in the interests of public safety, implying that if the suspension is not upheld, then public safety is at risk and deaths may ensue. With the spectre of this threat, no proof of justification needs to be offered – only an affirmation that an investigation is going on – and of course, this can go on for ages.

In an analysis of over 300 cases of suspension, less than 10 per cent were even remotely dangerous to the public. Many of the charges related to expenses, talking to the press, disobeying a Stasi or Trust policy; but once the shroud has been waved, it is difficult to get anyone to interfere, despite the consequences for the poor accused. What price public safety, after all? We have seen from what Stephen Thornton has said that the Stasi think of little else!

The European Court Of Human Rights

The argument that the United Kingdom has not yet integrated European Law into the British system is clearly now no longer tenable. A very good example of this was the issue about female service personnel being automatically dismissed from the military services if they became pregnant.[16] British military lawyers held that these dismissals were lawful and that Queen's Regulations[17] were paramount in these cases.

The European Court ruled otherwise. It deemed that sacking service women, just because they were pregnant, was discriminatory and therefore illegal. Substantial compensation was awarded. The supremacy of European Law is now accepted by the British legal system, and there are numerous other legal precedents to underline this.

If one tries to take a case to the European Court of Human

[16]This was once used as a means of leaving the service by ladies. It was always considered a cheaper option, however, to buy yourself out!

[17]The question will doubtless have come to the reader's mind: 'Is it fair to compare Queen's Regulations (which have formed the basis of military law for hundreds of years) with the misinterpretation of a few health circulars (HM 611/112; HC 90/9; and HSG 94/49) by a group of half-educated accountants?'

Rights in Strasbourg, then one has first to exhaust all possible local remedies, including going through the courts. The British legal system could thus be considered a (very expensive and time-consuming) stepping-stone. At the time of writing, there appears, however, to be some light at the end of the tunnel. Parliament has passed the Human Rights Bill. This means that:

> Trusts and Authorities which do not change their policies could be opening the floodgates for unlimited compensation claims, further draining NHS resources.[viii]

Dr Royce Darnell won a case in the European Court eleven (yes, eleven) years after he had been sacked from the Royal Infirmary in Derby in 1982. Nine judges ruled that the United Kingdom authorities were in breach of the Convention's guarantee to speedy recourse to justice!

Sadly, however, scrutiny of the Bill reveals that the Health Secretary will have the last word, and, in the past, holders of this office have been firmly on the side of the Stasi and 'the system'. Kafka-esque trials behind closed doors are likely to continue. Even when found innocent, the poor doctor may not be informed. A case has been recorded where a doctor hauled before a disciplinary tribunal was not informed that he had been found innocent for nine months (yes, nine months!). The reader will have to be assured that these Alice-in-Wonderland events are (sadly) true and have not been made up. Worse, during those nine months, the hospital authorities continually hinted that the decision had not gone in his favour. This was, of course, all part of the softening-up process before negotiating a settlement.

In another case, a suspension was maintained in spite of the fact that the hospital authorities knew that they could find nobody willing to say anything against the doctor. Nonetheless, he was subjected to a full enquiry into alleged personal misconduct – for speaking to the press (which contractually he was allowed to do). This proved to be part of a softening up process before negotiation of a settlement. It was only after this that he found out that no creditable witnesses against him could be found.

Normal legal procedure is to provide the accused with copies of all statements and allegations before the trial. If any of these are withdrawn, he should be notified. It would of course be unheard of for the court's decision not to be made available at once. *Normal* court procedure, however, is governed by ethics and driven by natural justice. This would not seem to be the case in the kangaroo courts of the NHS.

The Costs

It is established legal protocol that in a case which ends in a court action, the side that loses is legally bound to pay the other side's costs subject only to the judges discretion. In Industrial Tribunal cases each side is responsible for its own costs and there is no reimbursement, win or lose. Normally, allegations of professional misconduct or professional incompetence are dealt with by one of the medical protection societies – but none of these is bound contractually to defend the doctor. If the case is labelled personal misconduct (no matter how contrived such labelling may be), then the defence might be borne by the BMA (so long as the doctor is a member, and the Association agrees.)

Thus, it can be seen that cases occur where doctors have had to fund themselves. An advantage (probably the only one) is that control of the legal team is assured. The price for this can easily reach five, if not six, figures. Thus, bankruptcy (with consequent erasure from the Medical Register) is a very real risk.

A particularly nasty tactic is for the hospital, when their case looks like collapsing, to change the allegations. A new defence then has to be prepared against the new attack. The whole exercise can then be repeated. The reader may think that this is simply unbelievable. Think again. This happened four times[18] to one suspended doctor before the hospital grudgingly conceded that there was no case to answer. The hospital's cost were borne by the taxpayer – and it will come as no surprise to the reader that not one Stasi suffered.

It has been estimated that each suspension costs about half a million pounds, but, as there are so many costs to consider, it is difficult to arrive at any meaningful figure. The usual settlement terms seem to be eighteen months to two years of salary together with pension adjustments if possible. The pension rules state that a pension can be enhanced if the retirement is considered to be in the interest of the service; actuarially this is valued at about another year of salary. The Perth and Kinross Healthcare NHS Trust managed to spend an estimated £1 million on a suspended geriatrician in 1998. Some three years after sending her home (and paying her full salary to improve her garden) the Stasi hit on an innovative method to recoup their losses. The *Daily Mail* describes their cunning plan:

A Health Trust which has paid a suspended doctor £180,000 to sit at home is saving money by cutting patients' meals... Yesterday at lunchtime patients at Perth Royal Infirmary were told their meals were being cut. Instead of offering the regular three courses, these were limited to two. Patients will now have to choose either soup or a dessert to go with their main course.[ix]

---

[18]Yes, *four* times!

This particular unjustified exclusion went on for seven years.

The weekly newspaper for hospital doctors (imaginatively entitled *Hospital Doctor*!) ran a feature on suspensions and their (financial) cost.[x] Among the many horror stories was the case of a pathologist in Wales whose annual pay of £60,000 had been paid for four years. A locum had to be employed to do the work he should have been doing. On top of this were legal costs.... At the time this story was run, the case had still not been settled! However, as a result of it being aired, the Health Minister announced a review, which he said would focus on speeding up the processes involved. It should come as no surprise, with stories like this, that the annual bill to the NHS for 'disciplinary proceedings' runs into millions of pounds. The reader will no doubt readily acknowledge that this estimate only covers the simple financial burden – the pain and suffering and the invigoration of the compensation culture are not even considered.

No doctor has ever yet been successfully prosecuted because of the excessive beavering away by the Stasi ploughing through records dating back many years in a fruitless attempt to find evidence. It would seem reasonable, therefore, to have at least some form of time limit. There is otherwise no effective means of stopping this waste:

- the District Auditor who certifies the hospital accounts is in no position to judge whether a suspension is justified
- the National Audit Office and the Public Accounts Committee can only comment after the money has been spent.

The Outcomes

The Study Group of the Society of Clinical Psychiatrists has been collecting data on the suspension of senior hospital doctors for the past twenty years. Details are collated from the BMA and Medical Insurance societies and show that, up to 1996, the figures ran at about ten per annum. Following that they show a bizarre pattern of troughs and peaks, which appear to be directly related to prevailing political events. After the problems in cardiac surgery in Bristol publicised in 1998, suspensions rocketed; they underwent a ten-fold increase and continued to run at around ten a month for eighteen months. After this it suddenly dropped to only two in five months. This coincided with the run up to the General Election and its immediate aftermath. Following on the number gradually climbed back to a steady state of one suspension a month. Then suddenly in late 2006, it rose to almost five a month. This peak coincides with the MTAS (Medical Training Application Service) debacle, which was a disastrous plot by the Stasi that is universally acclaimed to be the worst example of medical mismanagement ever. It was a computerised attempt to prevent consultants allocating their house jobs to the most appropriate applicant (i.e. the person they wanted), and MTAS led to the brightest and most gifted young doctors in the country not getting a job when they qualified!

Reporting suspension to the Study Group is purely voluntary, although any mention 'on the grapevine' or in the media is always followed up. Not all doctors want to talk – they feel so deeply embarrassed that they simply want to hide; some have even committed suicide. Others are instructed by their employer not to talk, with the threat of increased disciplinary pressure if they do (especially to the media). Such talking is considered to bring the hospital into disrepute (as if there was anything to hide!). It is quite customary to have a gagging clause following settlements – not least for fear of the public's reaction to the waste of its own money.

The Study Group has data on 300 suspensions gathered over the past twenty years. Certain themes recur:

- Multiple charges can be made on a 'shotgun' principle to ensure a hit. Much is trivia – but it all contributes significantly to costs. For the analysis, the most serious charge was taken, together with whoever made it.
- By far the majority (309 out of 316 complete cases) were results of complaints which were not from patients. Of the seven (yes, only seven) complaints from patients, two were allegations of professional incompetence and only one of these was upheld.
- About a third were allegations of personal misconduct, but half the cases reported to the police for criminal investigation turned out to be unjustified.

One of the first actions of a hospital authority after suspending someone is to carefully go through claims such as travel expenses; as most doctors under-claim (or do not bother to claim at all) this rarely bears any fruit. In fact, police and Royal Automobile Club investigations following the suspension of a Welsh surgeon revealed that, far from cheating the authority, he was owed several thousand pounds. It became obvious that the original allegation had been made out of malice without any pretence at checking the facts. In another case where a consultant had been suspended 'for making a racial comment', his secretaries were questioned if he had ever had sex with them and the ward staff was asked if he had ever worn a 'Male Chauvinist Pig'[19] tie to work!

The Department of Health set up NCAS (National Clinical

---

[19]These ties, sadly no longer available, were usually bought by daughters, girlfriends and even wives and were quite popular in the 1970s. They were advertised in *Playboy* magazine on mail order. They featured a repeated design of a pink pig on either a blue or maroon background underneath which were emblazoned the letters MCP. When one of the authors wore one to work in the 1980s, he was asked if it stood for Manchester City Piggeries!

Advisory Service) which was supposed to have a system for sorting out which cases should be dealt with by an exclusion and of course it was agreed that exclusion would be reserved for the most exceptional circumstances. In little over a year after this system started, NCAS had more than 500 queries from Hospital Trusts to ask which doctors should be suspended.[xi] The *Apparatchiks*[20] could not make their own decisions.[21] As has been shown in the previous chapters, they have no formal training and as will have become apparent, they also lack initiative, intelligence and common sense.

Several doctors accused of misconduct have committed suicide.[22] The Study Group of the Society of Clinical Psychiatrists regard one of their greatest achievements to be that only one of those suspended doctors who had made contact with them had succumbed to this. The Group maintains a cross support service and has a national list of psychiatrists who can go to the help of a distressed doctor.

It seems bizarre that professional medical people attacked by their employer in this way have to be advised on how to protect

---

[20]*Apparatchik* is a Russian colloquial term for a full-time, professional functionary of the Communist Party or government; i.e., an agent of the party *apparat* (apparatus). Members of the *apparat* were frequently transferred between different areas of responsibility, usually with little or no actual training for their new areas of responsibility. The term was usually associated with a specific mindset, attitude and appearance of the person; when used by 'outsiders', it often bore derogatory connotations.

[21]In Dante's *Inferno*, the outermost circle of Hell is reserved for the indecisive.

[22]Clinical depression following suspension is common and should not be regarded as any indication of guilt. It seems to be related to the inability of the suspended doctor to cope with the threat to not only his livelihood but also his whole way of life – in addition to the bullying which we have described and which would not seem out of place in the former East European totalitarian regimes.

themselves from becoming fatally ill.[23] Private employers putting their staff in this situation would be prosecuted – but the NHS once again seems to be outside the law.

It is now considered that 'one in every fifty consultants is likely to be suspended at some point'! The reader may seek solace from the fact that this refers to consultants as a whole – the chance for the authors had always been somewhat higher, and thus for others, correspondingly lower!

The Nitty Gritty

Out of approximately one hundred cases of alleged professional incompetence (remember only seven came from patients i.e. 'customers'), in only twelve was a guilty verdict produced. This is despite the lighter burden of proof of simple *balance of probabilities* required.

Let us look more closely at those falsely accused. Ninety of the 116 accused by the Stasi were reinstated and the remainder had their contracts bought out and accepted a large financial settlement, because either the Stasi could not bear to face the humiliation of having to work with doctors whom they had falsely accused of wrongdoing, or the doctors themselves refused to continue to work at the same hospital, presumably fearing another knife in the back. Of the ninety-two accused by their medical colleagues, twenty-five had to have a financial settlement. The conclusion is that the Stasi were unable to

---

[23]Whilst on the subject of doctors dying, two of your authors have stipulated in their Last Will and Testament that they do not wish for any Stasis to attend their funeral services. The sad truth is that they won't take any notice and will still probably turn up and thus have the morning off work. The only consolation here (and that would be to surviving colleagues) is that it might prevent them doing further harm to patient care if they are kept away from the hospital!

control a situation whereby a colleague had accused a doctor of incompetence and this could not be upheld. The only way out was to negotiate a purchase of the contract. This represents a serious failure of management. It also represents a pretty poor hit rate – only one in five cases alleged by 'management' was made to stick and one in five did not return to work. This of course represents a serious wastage of highly skilled and experienced medical staff that the NHS can ill afford to lose. Remember, this is despite the marked bias of the whole procedure that has been amply demonstrated in 'We will get you, one way or another' (see above). Clearly, they are so incompetent, that they cannot even do this.

In contrast, the General Medical Council's disciplinary committee hearings (which are made public) find the majority of the accused guilty. This is despite a more difficult burden of proof, that of *beyond reasonable doubt*. Only two have been overturned following appeal to the Privy Council.

How can this be so? It is a widely held belief that doctors cover up for their colleagues and that no doctor will get another into trouble. It is clear that this is not the case – when it is necessary for disciplinary action to be taken, then the profession is ready to police itself – and, it is evident, with much more efficiency and expediency that the kangaroo courts of the Stasi.

Who Is Most At Risk?

Certain specialities appear to be more vulnerable. Pathologists seem particularly at risk and it seems to be because much of their work can be easily made available for detailed examination (histology slides are kept for years), yet, despite general feelings that it is entirely objective, it has a large degree of subjectivity. Surgeons as a whole are more vulnerable than physicians, and this could be because their work is more clearly interventionist. The most vulnerable specialty of all, however, are the obstetricians. It is always easy to allege that a stillborn child is the fault of the obstetrician and it is easier to make it stick if the obstetrician in question has had quarrels with some of his colleagues (irrespective of the facts). The Stasi, (who remember have absolutely no medical knowledge whatsoever) are scared stiff that there might just be some truth in the allegations and consider that the safest thing to do is to suspend the accused doctor and anyway this gives them a tremendous feeling of power over their intellectual betters. Remember, the vast majority of complaints are not brought by patients. Psychiatrists are vulnerable through their contact with other groups of staff (especially social services) and the trials of trying to care for patients in the community.

Regarding geographical location, West Midlands seems to be an especially risky area in which to practise medicine (more suspensions have occurred here than in whole regions elsewhere), followed by Wales. The study group has charted changes which have occurred when senior medical administrative staff have moved.

The Legality Of It All

One does not need legal training to realise that when it comes to the suspension of senior doctors, then the law (English, Scots and European!) has had a coach and horses driven through it. The law of contract demands that neither employer nor employee do anything to undermine the mutual trust and confidence that must exist between them. Of course, if this were followed to the letter, all the NHS hospitals would have to close down because almost all the consultants have absolutely no trust or confidence whatsoever in their incompetent administrative staff. Suspension upon flimsy grounds followed by a smear campaign necessarily undermines any trust which might have existed. That is not to say that suspension is never justified. Clearly, when the allegations are serious and adequately supported, a doctor should be suspended whilst the case is expeditiously investigated – by suitable independent expert bodies. This is the complete opposite of what usually happens, and it is small wonder that so many doctors, even when completely exonerated, feel unable to return to their job.

The Industrial Relations Act specifically requires staged warnings before dismissal. There should first of all be an oral warning, followed by a written warning and only finally should there be a disciplinary hearing. The Study Group could find no case (that is right, no case) where either an oral or written (let alone both) warning had been given to a doctor before suspension!

The nearest they came was an oral warning and counselling whilst the doctor and certain members of the Stasi met each other in a swimming pool! Indeed, one hospital authority claimed (or rather accepted the claim by its disciplinary panel) that it is not necessary to give these staged warnings to a doctor 'because the doctor is educated'.[24] Since this new 'case law' was made from a hearing conducted in secret, the reader will not get to know what degree of education has to be possessed to bar an educated person from the protection of the law.

The disciplinary process of the NHS breaks the European Convention of Human Rights on a massive scale. The relevant parts of Article 6 states:

---

[24]Apart from the primary implication that all should be treated equally before the law, this begs the question as to what constitutes 'education' – and how would these mandarins explain this to their other employees whom they obviously consider to be uneducated?

In the determination of his civil rights or of any criminal charge against him, everyone is entitled to a fair and public hearing within a reasonable time by an independent and impartial tribunal established by law. Judgment shall be pronounced publicly.

This is of major significance, and it is worth looking at each point more closely.

'Determination' is legalese for examination with a view to winding up or terminating.

'Civil rights' include the right to practise a well-established traditional profession which has its own code of conduct and system of maintaining standards, and which is necessary for economic independence. Case law from within the European Court has already established that to practise as a doctor is a civil right for those so recognised by the appropriate doctors' professional body (in the United Kingdom this is the GMC).

Suspension of a doctor clearly prevents him from following his profession. This is not only in the hospital from which he has been locked out, but also, it would seem, from all other NHS hospitals (and consequently private ones as well). Let us examine this total exclusion from practice. Hospital Trusts certainly prevent suspended doctors from doing locum posts in other Trusts. The justification for this is the old one of shroud waving – it is a pity that they do not expend so much energy on checking up on the details of the bogus doctors we from time to time read about. As we have seen, very few suspensions are in fact due to bad doctoring – perhaps they are trying to spare the public from further spurious travel claims, etc. It does make a mockery of the claim that suspension is a neutral process – it seems that anyone suspended is, by that very act, not only deemed guilty but also punished.

The practice of 'blacklisting'[25] is expressly against the advice in a book (written by two Administrators!) entitled *Disciplining and Dismissing Doctors in the National Health Service*. The relevant quotation is: 'It is perfectly in order for doctors to work elsewhere.'[xii] Many private hospitals also deny their facilities to doctors suspended by the NHS. The motive for this private sector exclusion could be the fear of losing trade, when on rare occasions the NHS have what they call an 'initiative' (to try to cut overlong waiting lists) and buy in private services.

It is amazing that the authority of the GMC can be flouted by such local arrangements and that the European Court of Human Rights ruling on civil rights counts for so little.

A 'fair and public hearing' is the entitlement of everyone, but the blatant violations of this have been quoted above. Let us look at the fairness issue first. It has always been a basic tenet of English (and Scots) law that one is deemed innocent until proven guilty. We have seen that the NHS has already discarded this. Perhaps the most outrageous recent contempt of the law has come in the White Paper from Sir Liam Donaldson in 2006, in which there is a move to alter the burden of proof necessary to dismiss a doctor from 'beyond reasonable doubt' to 'on the balance of probabilities'. European case law has already determined that the more severe the restraint enforced, the greater should be the burden of proof and here Sir Liam is suggesting that it should be reduced. Stripping a doctor of his civil right to practise his profession is clearly one of the most

---

[25]Black Lists were originally kept in Black Books and the original ones (compiled in the reign of Henry VIII to record the scandalous goings-on in monasteries) were bound in black leather! There were also Red Books and Blue Books. These black books must not be confused with Henry II's Black Books of the Exchequer.

severe sanctions that could ever be applied to him. Do we therefore assume that the NHS is just ignorant of the European Law or merely contemptuous of it? Sadly the truthful answer is that it is both! If this proposal goes through, one can envisage a steady stream of doctors appealing to the Court of Human Rights in Strasbourg and winning large sums of money, which the taxpayer has to pay, for the doctor's lost lifetime earnings because of this blatant abuse of his civil rights.

The NHS will doubtless bleat that this proposal is only to protect the public. The police also have a duty to protect the public but the criminal courts rightly demand that the burden of proof shall be beyond reasonable doubt and of course this still applies when life has been put at risk. English, Scots and Strasbourg courts all demand equality of arms in a fair fight: that means that lawyers of equal calibre slog it out together and each has the right to have his own expert witnesses. No such proposal exists for the NHS. Indeed in its disciplinary code, lawyers for the accused are allowed to attend but (amazingly) are not allowed to act in a legal capacity. Believe it or not, they are denied the right to cross-examine witnesses or challenge the evidence on behalf of the accused doctor. It was observed in the House of Commons that suspended doctors are treated worse than criminals.

In hospital secret tribunals, there is clearly no parity: both parties should have equal access to case notes[xiii] – this is difficult when the suspended doctor is denied access to the hospital! If we are going strictly 'by the book', then reports commissioned by the prosecution should be made available to both sides, including those that show the doctor in a favourable light. Suppression of such evidence is a further breach. Yet another infringement is the failure to reimburse costs. The Commission has ruled that the public nature of the proceedings helps to ensure a fair trial by protecting the litigant against arbitrary decisions and enabling society to control the administration of justice...

Let us now consider the second part of 'fair and public hearing'. There has been no 'public' hearing of a disciplinary tribunal involving a senior hospital doctor for more than twenty years.

'Within a reasonable time' sounds pretty straightforward, but as we have seen there have been suspensions lasting for ten years.

'By an independent and impartial tribunal'. Your authors realise that it sounds utterly incredible and reminiscent of former Iron Curtain regimes, but the reader is assured once again that members of the tribunal are chosen by the accusing health authority who also select the chairman from a list supplied by the Lord Chancellor's office. At least one health authority rejected several nominations of chairman from that list as they were 'not suitable'. Arguably, the chairman is in the hands of the health authority. 'Independent' should really mean independent of the Hospital Authority, rather than the accused. Nevertheless, one tribunal dismissed nearly forty witnesses because they were in favour of the doctor.

'Established by law'. The tribunal must be drawn from, appointed by, or answerable to the judiciary. The form of the tribunal must not be left to the discretion of the executive but must be left to legal regulation by Parliament[xiv] and have a legal basis. The General Medical Council is, the reader will be glad to learn, regulated by Parliament and directed under the jurisdiction of the highest court in the land, the Privy Council.[26]

'Judgment shall be announced publicly'. The normal practice of disciplinary inquiries against senior doctors is that the tribunal

---

[26]The reader is cautioned against assuming any connection with an outside lavatory.

reports to the Hospital Executive, giving its verdict directly to them. It does not tell the accused doctor, neither does it pronounce sentence.

It is clear that the hospital tribunal system against doctors is an antithesis of Article 6. It directly contravenes the European Convention of Human Rights, and is thus illegal under European Law. The most important facet is that these tribunals deny a doctor's civil right to follow his profession. Suspension alone is a breach and, because of the monopolistic nature of British medicine, is tantamount to being blacklisted. We are not suggesting that doctors should *never* be dismissed – but either the GMC or one of Her Majesty's Magistrates should only do that by due legal process. Any other suspension is illegal – and for those readers who collect such useful gems of information, the judgment is to be found in 6 EHRR 467 p583 Application No 10331/83 -v- United Kingdom.[27] For those Australian or American readers, EHRR is European Human Rights Report.

What About The Other Articles?

The reader is assured that this chapter will not simply cover the main crime of these self-appointed, embittered tyrants, serious though the breach of Article 6 is. There are also Articles 8 and 10.

Article 8: Everyone has the right to respect of his private and family life and his correspondence. There shall be no interference by a public authority with the exercise of this right except such as in accordance with law....

Although the Stasi (living up to their namesake, the East German

---

[27]Which in turn is based on 2EHRR, 170; and 4EHRR, 1!

Secret Police or *Staatssicherheitsdienst)* like to think that they are the law (and at times evidently that they are above the law), we have seen they are operating completely outside of it.[28] The tapping of telephones and interfering with the mail of doctors is clearly in contravention of Article 8.

> Article 10: Everyone has the right to freedom of expression. This right shall include freedom to hold opinions and to receive and impart information and ideas without interference by authority.

There are, of course, exclusions to this so that State secrets are protected and incitement to crime prevented. Article 10 also prevents slander of an individual or besmirching an individual's honour. Organisations, such as NHS Trusts, however, are not individuals and cannot be slandered. Indeed, Article 19 gives an individual the absolute right to criticise them at length. Nevertheless, four doctors have been suspended because they dared to talk to the press. They were all exonerated. That is not to say that they were restored to the position they were in before, even though they might have figuratively had 'no stain to their character'.

For those readers who may be averse to all this European Law stuff, the United Nations, in its Universal Declaration of Human Rights of 10 December 1948 covers exactly the same ground.[29]

---

[28]So far, however, the administrators have not shot any staff. On 15 August 2007 an order came to light in the voluminous *Ministerium für Staatssicherheit* (Stasi) archives ordering the East German Border Police to open fire on dissident Germans fleeing their wonderful Socialist State: the 1973 order said, 'Do not hesitate with the use of a firearm, including when the border breakouts involve women and children, which the traitors have already frequently taken advantage of.'

[29]The relevant articles are: Articles 7, 8, 10, 12 and 19.

How About a Quick Trip to Continental Europe?

Before one embarks on the journey to Strasbourg for a legal remedy, there are some very strict rules, which must be considered. The exact details of the procedure are to be found in every public library.[30] The most important thing to bear in mind is that all local remedies (courts etc) must have been exhausted and that the submission to Strasbourg must be within six months of the final exhaust (amazing how one falls into their jargon). The present attempts to incorporate the European Convention into the British legal system should result in fewer cases having to go to Johnny Foreigner. It should mean that some disputes (particularly where there is no legal precedent) could be dealt with quickly in the United Kingdom. This is what happens in most other European countries. There are currently more cases against the UK heard in Strasbourg than against any other country.

Natural Justice

There is another area of law, which is also regularly broken in these disciplinary cases. This concerns the Tribunals of Inquiry Act 1921 and the rules of natural justice. It is an important area, but like so many aspects of the law, tedious and boring. Nevertheless, the detail is reproduced here for completeness. Now might be a good time to take a short break, especially if the reader has so far (like the majority) read to this page without putting the book down.

The situation was admirably described in the Normansfield inquiry; this concerned itself with the performance, behaviour and conduct of staff at Normansfield Hospital. The dispute was

---

[30]And, who knows, perhaps these days on the Internet. The authors do not know.

between the Chief Psychiatrist and the para-medical staff over the management of patients.

Para 13: In view of the fact that many professional reputations were at stake and grave questions of integrity and good faith were likely to arise, we were determined to put into operation the safeguards of the rules of natural justice: what has been described as 'fair play in action'. We took as our yardstick the recommendations of the report of the Royal Commission on Tribunals on Inquiry of which Lord Justice Salmon (now Lord Salmon of Sandwich) was Chairman[31] (Command 3121, November 1966). The main rules of fairness suggested therein and accepted by the Government (Command 5313, 1973) are:

   i Before any person become involved in an Inquiry, the Tribunal must be satisfied that there are circumstances which affect him and which the Tribunal proposes to investigate.
   ii Before any person who is involved in an Inquiry is called as a witness; he should be informed of any allegations, which are made against him and the substance of the evidence in support of them.
   iii (a) He should be given adequate opportunity of preparing his case and of being assisted by legal advisers.
   (b) His legal expenses should normally be met out of public funds.
   iv He should have the opportunity of being examined

---

[31]Note, he was not the 'Chair'.

by his own Solicitor or Counsel and of stating his case
in public at the Inquiry.

v Any material witness he wishes called at the Inquiry
should, if reasonably practicable, be heard.

vi He should have the opportunity of testing by cross
examination conducted by his own Solicitor or Counsel
any evidence, which may affect him.

They also took their level of proof that the evidence should be
serious and have weight and substance that matches any serious
charge or outcome. This definition is beyond 'the balance of
probabilities', but does not reach quite as far as 'beyond all
reasonable doubt'. When there is the possibility of dismissal, the
evidence should exclude trivia and natural justice demands that it
should be substantial and well beyond the balance of probabilities.

Because of the important precedent of this Normansfield
Hospital case and the very clear 'main rules of fairness suggested
therein', all hospital disciplinary tribunals should take this lead
and follow the fairly straightforward rules of natural justice.

Sadly, this is not the case and successive tribunals since then
have broken these rules.

The General Medical Council

The ethical code of the GMC is very detailed as to how doctors
should behave. They should not make disparaging comments
about medical colleagues. Obviously, if there is a belief that a
colleague is breaking the law, then there is a duty to inform the
authorities. If it is thought that performance is not up to scratch,
then the doctor is ethically bound to discuss this with the
underperforming colleague – there may be extenuating clinical
circumstances. If that fails, then discussion should include other

medical colleagues, with the possibility of the GMC being approached for action. In this way, the public is protected, and no rights violated.

The Stasi do also have a code – unhappily, it is a rather vague wish list, with seemingly no means of appropriate enforcement. A proper profession demands ethical rules and means by which they may be enforced. Perhaps one day this happy state of affairs may be achieved – at present doctors (good and bad) seem to be fair game for anybody who, supported by the public purse, wants to 'have a go'.

CONCLUSION

The NHS is definitely very sick.

It is very likely, in the opinion of many British Hospital Consultants,[i] that it is terminally ill and might soon be in its death throes! If something radical is not done in the very near future, it will certainly not be able to continue to exist as we know it.

The cause of this illness is that it has a huge cancerous growth inside, sapping it of all its strength. That malignant mass is the Management System. The analogy to a cancer is apt. A patient with cancer does not know for quite a long time that a disease is present: the vast majority of the British public is utterly unaware of the true cause of the sickness of the NHS.

Another characteristic of a tumour to a pathologist is that 'it grows at the expense of the healthy tissues around it without at the same time serving any useful function': that could not be truer. To the detriment of the professionals, administration has grown bigger and bigger and it has certainly not served any useful purpose. Quite the reverse. The anecdotes in the book prove that beyond all reasonable doubt. Most intelligent clinicians believe that the administrators are so useless, it would be better if they were paid to stay at home! But they are worse than that; just like a tumour, their presence is actually harmful to one's wellbeing.

A tumour starts off with a few abnormal cells, which then go on proliferating beyond normal control. It grows and grows until it sometimes becomes bigger than the organ from which it has arisen. Cancer can eventually kill its host by an insidious process of infiltration and spread. The administrators have certainly done this. Twenty years ago there was just a handful, but now there are countless numbers of them. By their own exorbitant salaries and continuing mismanagement and misuse of money, they have diverted precious funds and have made our once thriving Health Service into an emaciated shadow of its former self. Sometimes cancer causes haemorrhage or bleeding. Then the blood flows away and cannot be replaced quickly enough by the ailing body. Doctors and nurses (the life blood of the NHS) have been leaving (or taking early retirement) in unprecedented numbers. And they are going because of the administration, which has made them feel absolutely and utterly unvalued.

The only treatment for a cancer is to completely get rid of it.

In the prolegomenon of this book, it was pointed out that if all (yes, every last one!) of the managers were to be sacked, the overall effect would be in an improvement of the service. This change for the better would result from the immediate and overwhelming increase in morale not only of the doctors and nurses but of everyone else in the hospital, who would be overjoyed at getting rid of the hated 'managers'. The importance of morale in a large corporate organisation such as a hospital is enormous. In addition to this, of course would be the immense savings. It was pointed out in the prologue that sacking every last one was not a serious proposal and that perhaps half a dozen administrators be retained by the larger hospitals, but that they were kept firmly under the control of clinical staff.

In the first chapter, Albert Schweitzer's self evident truth about the importance of doctors in running a hospital was invoked: you cannot run a hospital without doctors – but you sure as hell can run one without administrators. The age-old lie is wheeled out over and over again, that since Schweitzer's days, things have changed and 'the doctor is different, the patient is different, and the medicine is different'.

Technology is cited as a cause for needing managers. However, it has been effectively shown that the administrators know nothing about technology. The sad truth is they know nothing about medicine, they know nothing about nursing; they know absolutely nothing at all about leadership: unfortunately, they do not even know about civil service administrative procedures. As always, your authors will be generous and say that perhaps they once knew something about double-entry bookkeeping!

In 2007, management guru, Sir Gerry Robinson was set a challenge by the BBC.[1] He went to work in an NHS Hospital (in Rotherham) for six months to try to help reduce the waiting lists. As an outsider, his first impression was surprise at the 'power struggle' between doctors and managers. He left 'with a very frustrated feeling that actually quite small sums of money properly and sensibly spent could have produced very large results in terms of reduced waiting lists, and actually very large sums of money had been thrown at the NHS and produced very little'. When Gordon Brown replaced Tony Blair as Prime Minister

---

[1] It was called 'Can Gerry Robinson Fix the NHS?'

in June 2007, Sir Gerry gave the new PM some public advice. He pointed out that the staggering amounts of money (around £90 billion) thrown at the NHS should really have improved the service but that 'sadly and quite frankly', it had not. He then said that what the NHS really needed was some 'really good managers.'

But where will they find them? And who on Earth will appoint them? Surely not other wholly untrained and woefully incompetent management colleagues?

Sadly and quite frankly, really good managers just do not seem to exist in the NHS.˝

Experience over the last twenty years has shown administrative fiasco after fiasco. What was once the envy of the world has been sadly degraded by these bureaucrats and left with feelings of hopelessness and despair. In 2007, morale was said to be 'so low that doctors would not recommend a medical career to family or friends'.ⁱⁱ Perhaps the most amazing question, however, is how did the degradation of the NHS and its doctors ever come about? How could the evil system infiltrate our health service, and then suspend a hospital consultant for eleven years without even telling him what his fault was? How on earth did these people with no prior knowledge of medicine or hospitals then get into positions of great power?

It has been shown in the last chapter to what extents of abuse they have misused this authority. Why though were they ever allowed to put themselves outside the law and convene kangaroo courts in which they chose not only the judge, but the jury, and then amazingly reserved the right whether or not to accept the verdict?

Certainly the whole issue around the suspension of doctors must be brought to public attention and changed by Parliament as soon as possible. Apart from the unbelievable inhumanity and unfairness of it all, it is wasting millions of pounds of taxpayers' money. Statistics for 2006 showed that it is not unusual for around 100 doctors to be suspended at any one time and with the average length of suspension between one and a half and two years, it was projected that the total bill to the Health Service is between £20million and £25million per year. Clearly this misuse of funds and the NHS manager's absolute disregard for natural justice must be stopped and the sooner the better.

It was so much fairer in the days of self regulation and a Tribunal of three very senior hospital consultants ('Three Wise Men'). If the main criticism of the old system is that it was too one-sided, then surely this same criticism is now even more valid: from the examples in the last chapter the reader may have been convinced that it is at present much more biased than three colleagues ever were. And in addition it is against all the principles enshrined in British Justice. It is totally unjust.

Remorse is one of the most destructive of emotions – you can never go back to alter things, and doctors know that they must shoulder a large part of the blame for this revolution.

> British doctors failed to notice that the world around them had changed utterly.... Doctors seemed to think that they were still living in Gladstone's world of minimal government, benign self-regulation, and a self-effacing state.[iii]

Doctors failed to realise what Draconian changes the administrators would enforce – even putting themselves outside the law to humiliate consultants – and now it all seems too late. One of the most disturbing features is that there appears to be no solution; there is no going back. Not only medicine but also the whole of society has changed. The replacement of professionalism by managerialism has overthrown a system which had slowly developed over generations. Moreover, during that process of evolution it had blossomed and improved. Thirty years ago, doctors had an ethos of duty – and with that duty went a degree of privilege. Patients on the whole would respect their medical attendants: it went without saying; they would, however, implicitly expect their doctor to make a visit in the middle of the night if necessary – that too went without saying. There was an old fashioned *Boy's Own Paper* sense of chivalry.

Sadly, that professionalism has now been dismantled and what is perhaps saddest of all is that, like Vesalius in his sixteenth century anatomy theatre, it is we doctors who have been duped into dismembering it! If we had only shown solidarity in the 1980s, and just refused to have anything to do with them; if in effect we had not collaborated.[2] They appealed to our baser instincts and offered financial incentives: we prostituted ourselves and took the bait. It is now far too late to take united action against them, and besides, doctors will never all agree now to present a united front – they are far too individualistic.

Nevertheless, if we all said in one voice, we would no longer collaborate, cooperate or communicate with hospital administrators, they could do absolutely nothing without us.

But it will never happen. All consultants can look around their

---

[2] In France during, and after, World War II, collaborators had their heads shaven and were branded on the scalp with the sign of a swastika; in Northern Ireland, during the Troubles, colleens who collaborated with British soldiers were similarly shorn, then stripped and tied to lamp-posts where they were tarred and feathered (a punishment first accorded to thieves on Crusaders' boats). Your authors would not of course suggest that all medical directors should suffer this indignity: suffice it that they are branded as wilfully treacherous individuals devoid of all moral worth and totally unfit to be received into the society of worthy men who prize honour and virtue above the external advantages of rank and fortune.

hospitals and pick out the Quislings – the lickspittles willing to sell their Hippocratic values for a merit award. There will always be the sycophantic turncoat who will put filthy lucre before his duty to his patients and take on the job of medical director. Yet anyone who applies for a job as medical director 'to represent his colleagues' is by definition inappropriate for that post: the type of consultant who is interested in taking on this office is clearly not a true representative of his colleagues, or he would not apply!'[3]

What seems so unspeakably sad is that there is no going back for another try. When we started to work for the NHS around twenty-five years ago, it was all so different. Hospitals then were happy places to work in. People got on with each other. There were no managers! Doubtless, the finances then were in as bad a state as they are now, but everybody had great morale. We all pulled together and had a sense of *esprit de corps*, of belonging; and an old-fashioned ethic of duty that we would work long hours, for poor rewards and all for the good of our patients. The old system had been built up from years and years of tradition which pre-dated Bevan's health service. Now it has been dismantled, and it would be impossible to even start to put it back together again.

Putting doctors into permanent management jobs does not even seem to be the answer. In the past, the drain sniffers had all the power, but then as now, administration seemed to attract the least skilful doctors, who for this same reason were not accorded with a high degree of respect from their peers. Indeed, according to one of your author's older colleagues, hospital administration seemed a particularly attractive career option to the least hardworking practitioners who did not cherish the prospect of

---

[3] This is sometimes known as a Catch-22 situation.

long hours working with patients, being on call, and visiting poorly folk in the middle of the night.[4] More recently, the motives of those doctors who have chosen to collaborate with the administrators are not infrequently interpreted (by those doctors who choose to spend more of their working time with their patients) as pecuniary and traitorous.

Perhaps an ideal solution would be that a newly retired consultant, respected and elected by his peers (i.e. other medically qualified consultants at that same hospital) should be appointed for a finite term of office (certainly no longer than a period of three years). The Ancient Greeks realised that if one person is in power for too long, things start to go badly wrong.[5] He need not be full time: indeed, it would be much better if he only went in for a few hours a week to sort things out (preferably just before they went wrong). He would have the absolute respect of everyone in the hospital and also the community. He would have the personal experience of many years of hospital work and above all he would be a *doctor* with all that implies. Physicians are usually highly intelligent and hard-working individuals, who place the wellbeing of the patients who have entrusted themselves into their care above all other considerations, particularly those of money and financial reward. They have served the whole of their working life with that ethic in the forefront of their minds. On the whole and even in the twenty-first century, society still respects its doctors.

Your authors cannot claim that this is a completely new and

---

[4]His actual words were: 'Spit on one drain-sniffer, and you'd drown 'em all'.

[5]The Greeks had Pericles; we have had Mr Blair (and Mrs Thatcher).

innovative idea conceived by them. This practical working solution for an almost insoluble problem had a forerunner in the pre-Bevan days, when a very senior and well-respected consultant was appointed by his colleagues as Medical Superintendent. He was not retired from his clinical consultancy in those days, however: he was still busy working. He would certainly have shunned any reference to that odious and demeaning term 'manager' and was too busy with his medical work to do any administering (even if he'd wanted to); his role was to help out and advise the Hospital Secretary (you may remember he was the shabbily-dressed harassed-looking cove in a crumpled suit). The Hospital Secretary was employed wholly and exclusively to administer and resource clinical decisions made by the consultants, and he knew his place.

Undoubtedly the critics would say that any suggestion of re-appointing a Medical Superintendent would be 'turning the clock back over fifty years!' Perhaps so, but it would be going back to a time when people were glad to work in hospitals, in which in turn were efficient, clean and happy places to work. It would be a return to a time when doctors trusted other members of the hospital staff and felt respected and valued by the community in which they worked. They might even stop retiring years before their time!

It is sad the clock cannot be turned back to this excellent system of hospital management, but as the poet once said:

The Moving Finger writes; and having writ,
Moves on: nor all thy Piety or Wit
Shall lure it back to cancel half a Line,
Nor all thy Tears wash out a Word of it.[iv]

POSTLEGOMENON

In a paper sent out by the British Association of Otolaryngologists (head and neck surgeons), there is a telling line:

> It is better to write to somebody who can do something about a problem rather than endlessly relate it to those who cannot.

It is tempting to recount (often at great length) problems one has encountered and in doing so, bore those who might well have been able to put things right, or at least be sympathetic to one's plight. It is also easy, once one has started, to 'get into a groove' – especially when one has established a reputation in that field. Many pundits continue when they have little new to say, and one should perhaps be mindful of that great English physician, Thomas Sydenham. He was sixty-four when his final work appeared. He ended by admitting that he had no more to say on his subject and that he had written everything he knew about medicine. He died with no further comments in print.

REFERENCES

Chapter 1

i Report on the Sanitary Conditions of the Labouring Population of Great Britain, 1842.

ii First Report on the Joint Working Party of the Organisation of Medical Work in Hospitals. London: HMSO, 1967. p3.

iii Turner S. 'Consultants prepare to fight off title challenge,' *BMA News Review* 1996;1:26-27.

iv Jones W H S. *Greek Medical Etiquette*. Ann Med Hist 1924; 6:138.

v D'Irsay S. *The Evolution of the Physician's Attitude*. Ann Med Hist 1928;10:376-386.

vi Jayne W A. *Healing Gods of Ancient Civilization*. New Haven, 1925. p 104.

vii Marett R R. *Psychology and Folklore*. London: Routledge, 1920. p217.

viii Dittrick H. *Fees in Medical History*. Ann Med Hist 1928; 10:90-101.

ix McLoughlin. *The Medical Profession and Medical Reform in Ireland 1830 - 1858*. Presentation at Symposium *Aspects of Nineteenth Century Irish Medical History* Dept. Modern History National University Ireland Maynooth 9 May 1998.

x Granshaw L. *Fame and fortune by means of bricks and mortar: the medical profession and specialist hospitals in Britain, 1800-1948*. In: Granshaw L, Porter R (eds) *The Hospital in History*. London: Routledge, 1989.

xi Barclay J. *In Good Hands: the History of the Chartered Society of Physiotherapy 1894-1994*. London: Butterworth Heinemann, 1994.

xii Larkin G. *The emergence of para-medical professions*. In: Bynum W F, Porter R (eds) *Companion Encyclopaedia of the History of Medicine*. London: Routledge, 1993 vol 2, pp1329-1349.

Chapter 2

i Montgomery of Alamein. *History of Warfare*. London: Collins, 1968. p27.

ii Ibid p22.

iii Ibid p23.

iv Keep P. *Penny Pinchers are Killing Staff Morale*. Hospital Doctor 1997; 17 July, p24-26.

v Grange J. *Take Morale Stance*. Hospital Doctor 1997; 17 July, p24.

vi Stephen H. *Complaints System a Cause for Concern*. Hospital Doctor 19 Jun 1997, p14.

vii Norman Muir, Editor *Just Another Monday? The 50th Anniversary of the National Health Service*. Glasgow: MDDUS, 1988.

viii Lee Potter J. *A Damn Bad Business*. London: Gollancz, 1977. p28.

ix Lord Nolan. *Standards in Public Life*. London: HMSO, 1995.

x Hunt G. *Whistleblowing in the Health Service, Accountable Law and Professional Practice*. London: Edward Arnold, 1995.

xi Craft, N. *Secrecy in the NHS*. Br Med J 1994;309:1640-1643.

xii Personal letter: Minister of State to M.P. POH (2) 5131/56 of 1998.

xiii Albert Einstein (reported in Weeks D, James, J. *Eccentrics* London: Weidenfeld & Nicholson, 1995 p63).

xiv Armstrong M. *White Paper Points the Way to Quality*. BMA News Review 1998; Jan, p3.

xv Mansfield A O. *Hospital Practice*. J Roy Soc Med 1998; 91: Supplement 36, p14-17.

xvi Medicopolitical Digest. Br Med J 1998; 317:1161.

xvii Appleby L. *A Medical Tour through the whole Island of Great Britain*. London: Faber and Faber, 1994.

xviii Wallace M., Berlin A. *Dropouts from London medical schools: a comparison with the rest of the United Kingdom*. Health Trends. 1997/98; 29(4):106-108.

xix Times 18 June 1998, p15.

xx Editorial: *Boomers would pay to simplify*. USA Today 7 Nov 1997, p1.

xxi News in Brief. Hospital Doctor 2 July 1998, p40.

Chapter 3

i Carmalt, W.H. *Address of the President*. Transactions of the American Surgical Association 1908;26:1-14 [page 9].

ii Jefferies I. *It Wasn't Me!* Harmonsworth: Penguin, 1969 p9.

iii Kriegel L. *Falling into Life*. In: Carmichael A G, Tatzan R M (ed) *Medicine. A Treasury of Art and Literature*. New York: Hugh Lauter Levin Assoc., 1991.

REFERENCES

iv Lord Horder. Forward in Herbert S M. *Britain's Health*. Pelican.

v Department of Health & Social Security *NHS 20th Anniversary Conference*. HMSO, 1968.

vi Lee Potter, J. 1997 *op. cit.* p31.

vii Griffiths R. *NHS Management Inquiry Report*. HMSO, 1983.

viii Webster C. *The National Health Service - A Political History*. Oxford, 1998.

ix Bruggen P. *Who Cares? True Stories of NHS Reforms*. Carpenter, 1997. p5.

x Enthoven A. *Reflections on the Management of the NHS*. Occasional Paper 5. London: Nuffield Hospitals Trust, 1985.

xi Br Med J 1989;299:756.

xii Kelly J. *A Complete Collection of Scottish Proverbs*. 1721.

xiii Lee-Potter 1997 *op.cit.* p123.

xiv Lee-Potter 1997 *op. cit.* p123.

xv Macbeth, Act 1 scene 7, ll 1-2.

xvi *Ex-Admiral claims sex-discrimination by NHS*. The Herald 4 September 1993, p2.

xvii *Admiral Wins Damages For Sex Bias Over Health Post.* Daily Telegraph. 22 November 1993, p6.

Chapter 4

i Strong A. *Badges Can't Take Place Of A Uniform (letter). Nursing Standard* 1998;13(3):11.

ii Fletcher R. *Nurse Row Goes On.* Hospital Doctor. 15 January 1998, p25.

iii Watson C. *Nurse Role Row Goes On.* Hospital Doctor. 15 January 1998, p25.

iv Mascie-Taylor H. *Where Is The Power Now*? Clinician In Management 1998;7(1):24.

v Williams D I. *The past: "the good old days".* J.Roy.Soc.Med. 1998;91: Supplement 36, p5-7.

vi Daily Mail Weekend magazine 8 August p8.

vii Editorial: *Nurse to Doctor Medical Upgrade* BMA News Review Aug 1998, p17.

viii Anon. Personal Communication. August 1998.

ix Thomson A. *Sister Pat "Is Not Shunned".* Plymouth Herald 22 December 1994.

REFERENCES

x Thomson A. *Sister Pat Shunned*. Plymouth Herald 17 December 1994.

xi Walsh J. *Nursing Sister Told To Leave Work*. Plymouth Herald 6 May 1994

xii Walsh J. *Support For Nursing Sister*. Plymouth Herald 10 May 1994.

xiii Herald Reporters. *Sacking Of Nurse Backed By 25 Sisters*. Plymouth Herald 20 August 1994.

xiv Walsh J. *Official Tries To Bar Sacked Nurse Demo*. Evening Herald 25 August 1994.

xv Thomson A. *Sister Pat Shunned*. Plymouth Herald. 17 December 1994.

xvi Nuki P. *Health Board Spent £200,000 on £34 Feud*. The Sunday Times 22 February 1998 p4.

xvii Anon. Personal Communication. September 1998.

xviii Bruggen , Peter *op. cit.* p. 212.

*xix Ibid.*p.215.

Chapter 5

i G B Shaw: *The Socialist Criticism of the Medical Profession*. Paper read to the Medico Legal Society 16 February 1909.

ii G B Shaw. Preface on Doctors. In *The Doctor's Dilemma*. 1906

iii Jefferies I. *It Wasn't Me!* Harmonsworth: Penguin, 1969 p87-88.

iv Personal communication 4 March 1997.

v Personal communication 27 March 1997.

vi Chaucer G. *Canterbury Tales* (1430) Prologue ll 443-444.

vii Hammond E A. *Incomes of Medical English Doctors*. J Hist Med 1960; Apr: 156.

viii D'Arcy Power. *The Fees of our Ancestors*. Lancet 1909;i:339-340.

ix Pericles, v i.

x Janus. Harlem: De Groen F Bohn. 1909

xi St Clair Thompson. *Annual Oration*. Medical Society of London 1916, p263.

xii Mehrotra T N. Fair System Of Remuneration. *Hospital Doctor* 10 June 1999 p26.

xiii Address, *Annual Meeting Association Surgeons in Training*, 1994.

xiv Cornford F M. *Microcosmographia Academica*. Cambridge: Bowes & Bowes, 1908 p19.

Chapter 6

i Masha, O. *Juniors Demand Free Car Parking*. Hospital Doctor 10 June 1999, p9.

ii BBC NEWS:http://news.bbc.co.uk/go/pr/fr/-/1/hi/health/4850562.stm.Published: 2006/03/28 05:04:28 GMT

iii BBC NEWS:http://news.bbc.co.uk/go/pr/fr/-/1/hi/health/4853084.stm.Published: 2006/03/28 13:10:41 GMT

iv Arribas E, Gasllardo C, Molina M. *Noise Contamination in the Public Hospital of Albacete. Noise as a Public Health Problem.* Proceedings Noises and Man '93 - 6th International Congress 1993; 2:331-333.

v Bisio G, Magrini A. *Acoustic Survey Of The Noise Levels In A Middle Size Town - The Influence Of Some Traffic Restrictions.* Proc Internoise 92, Toronto 1991 July 20-22.

vi Bergland B, Lindvall T. *Community noise*. Archives of the Center for Sensory Research 1995; 2:1-195.

vii Spiers J. *The Invisible Hospital and the Secret Garden - An Insider's Commentary on the NHS Reforms.* Radcliffe Medical Press, Oxford: 1995. p185.

viii BMA News Review August 1994 p19.

ix Pelling M. *Medical practice in early modern England: trade or profession*? In: Prest W (ed) *The professions in early modern England*. London: Croom Helm, 1987 p104.

x Ueyama T. *Capital, Profession and Medical Technology: The Electro-Therapeutic Institutes and the Royal College of Physicians, 1888-1922*. Medical History 1997; 41:150-181.

xi Larson M. *The rise of professionalism: a sociological analysis*. Berkeley and Los Angeles: University of California Press, 1977.

xii Pelling M. *Occupational diversity: barbersurgeons and the trades of Norwich, 1550-1640*. Bull Hist Med 1982;56:484-511.

xiii Reader W. *Professional men: the rise of the professional classes in nineteenth-century England*. London: Weidenfeld & Nicolson, 1966.

xiv Waddington I. *General practitioners and consultants in early nineteenth-century England: the sociology of an intra-professional conflict*. In: Woodward J, Richards D (eds) *Health care and popular medicine in the social history of medicine*. New York: Holmes & Meier, 1977.

xv Digby A. *Making a medical living: doctors and patients in the English market for medicine, 1720-1911*. Cambridge: Cambridge University Press, 1994.

xvi Johnson, Samuel. Boswell. *Life*.vol 3, page 19. (5th April 1776) *xvii* Quinn F B. *Epistaxis: A Safe Treatment Plan. Lecture* delivered at 28th Annual Otolaryngology Conference, Galveston 1997.

xviii George Bernard Shaw. Preface on Doctors. In: *The Doctor's Dilemma*, 1906.

xix Hodges R E L. *Home Guard Medical.* Bulletin Military Historical Society 1998; 48:135.

Chapter 7

i Loudon I. *Words: Nosocomial.* Br Med J 1998; 317:1242.

ii Burchfield R. *The English Language.* Oxford: Oxford University Press, 1985. p109.

iii Personal communication.

iv Andrews E. *Medical Terminology.* Ann Med Hist 1923; 10:195.

v Personal communication.

vi Wyld H C W. *Universal Dictionary of the English Language.* London: Waverly, 1957 9th ed p205b.

vii Personal communication.

viii Personal communication.

ix Personal communication.

x Personal communication GMC/DL/7083 28 October 1997.

xi Cunliffe R J. *Blackie's Compact Etymological Dictionary.* Glasgow: Blackie, 1920.

xii Dooling R. *Critical Care* London: Pan, 1992. p161.

xiii Editorial The Practising Midwife 1998; 1:45.

Chapter 8

i Tomlin, P.J. *The Suspensions Scandal.* J Obstetrics & Gynaecology, 2003; 23(3):221-217.

ii Morris Z. Hospital Doctor 27 October 1998, p17.

iii Hawler P. Hospital Doctor. 29 October 1998, p39.

iv Milburn, A. (1995) *The Suspension of Dr O'Connell.* Committe of Public Acounts Report No. 40. London. HMSO

v Donaldson, L.J. (1994) *Doctors with problems in an NHS work force.* Brit Med J 308: 1277-1282

vi North Devon Journal 21 June 2007 p. 1.

vii Hospital Doctor *Ibid* p40.

viii Morris Z. *Europe last hope in fight for rights.* Hospital Doctor 29 October 1998. p16.8

REFERENCES

ix Currie, G. (1998) *Trust dishes out cuts.* Daily Mail 22 July page 26.

x Morris Z. *Senior Suspension Becomes An Epidemic.* Hospital Doctor 29 October 1998. p32-33.

xi Andrews, Baroness (2003) *Doctors: Suspension.* Hansard. 19 March, Col 234. London. HMSO.

xii Bunbury T, McGregor A. *Disciplining And Dismissing Doctors In The National Health Service.* Mercia Publications, 1988.

xiii van Dijk P, Hoof G J H. *Theory and Practice of the European Convention on Human Rights.* 2nd ed, p320.

xiv van Dijk P, Hoof G J H. *Theory and Practice of the European Convention on Human Rights.* 2nd ed, p339

Conclusion

i Taylor, K. *Bringing Managers to Book for what They Do.* Hosp. Doctor, 20 July 2006, page 26.

ii Medicine *"a Bad Job" Say Gloomy Doctors.* Editorial 12 April 2007, page 1.

iii Editorial. *Core Values.* Br Med J 1995; 309:1247-1248.

iv Fitzgerald E. *The Rubáiyat of Omar Khayyám.* (1st ed) Verse 51.